Welcome to Medic Mind!

Dear School Leaders,

Firstly, let us introduce ourselves. Medic Mind is a UK-based company, set up in July 2017, with the aim of helping students with all aspects of their medical applications. Since then, we have continued to grow in strength and expertise, adding five more support programmes: Vet Mind, Dentist Mind, Law Mind, Oxbridge Mind and Study Mind.

Over the years, we have supported more than **55,000** students in pursuing their educational dreams and have partnerships with over **100** schools and institutions including Eton College, Queen Elizabeth's Grammar School and Oxford International College.

We hope that both you and your students benefit from the textbooks we have sent you. Please have a look through our brochure to find out more about our services and how we can help you further support your students through their educational journey.

Yours faithfully,

Dr Mohil Shah and Dr Kunal Dasani
Medic Mind Founders

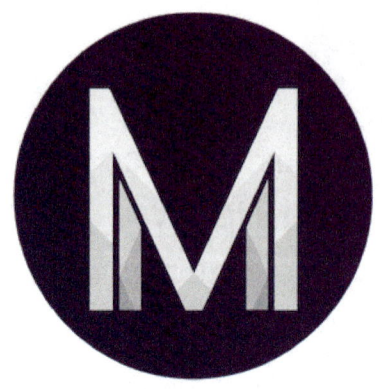

MEDIC MIND

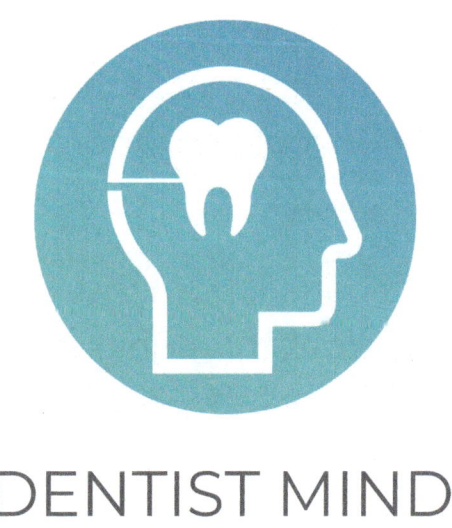

DENTIST MIND

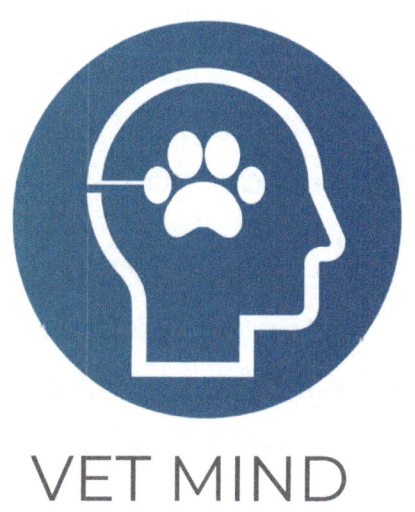

VET MIND

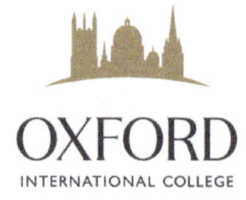

Jason Brooks
Oxford International College

We have been working with Medic Mind for 3 years in the upskilling of our students for top university destinations for medicine. We have always found the services provided by Medic Mind commendable. The management team of Medic Mind has always taken care of our company's requirements and the needs of our students. They have always shown great patience and professionalism. I truly appreciate Medic Mind's work. So, I strongly support the recommendation for Medic Mind to be considered part of your supply chain.

Medic Mind in a Nutshell

Medic Mind provides high-quality school programmes for a range of different subject types. Our key highlights:

- **Industry leaders -** leaders in 1-1 tutoring with experienced tutors and established courses.

- **Reputation for Quality -** ranked in TrustPilot's Top 4 UK Tutors with thousands of 5* reviews.

- **Standardised Materials** - students are provided with online courses, question banks and video tutorials, all created by our in-house academic team.

- **Trusted School Partners** - working directly with universities and schools to provide high quality lessons. Partner schools include: Oxford International, Eton College, Cardiff Sixth Form College, King's College London and Bristol University.

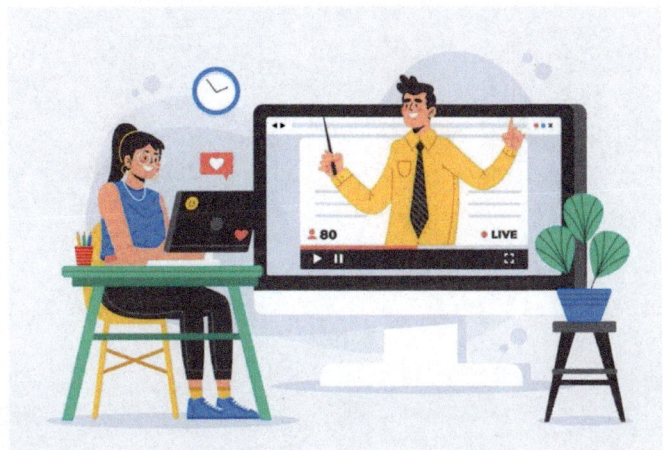

What does Medic Mind provide in their UCAT + BMAT Packages?

An engaging and interactive Classroom Day

We will come to your school and provide the ultimate crash course in the UCAT and BMAT by teaching your students everything they need to know to ace the test!

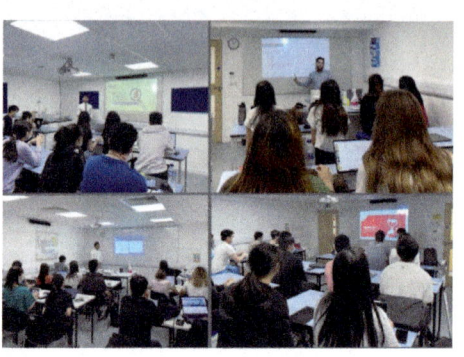

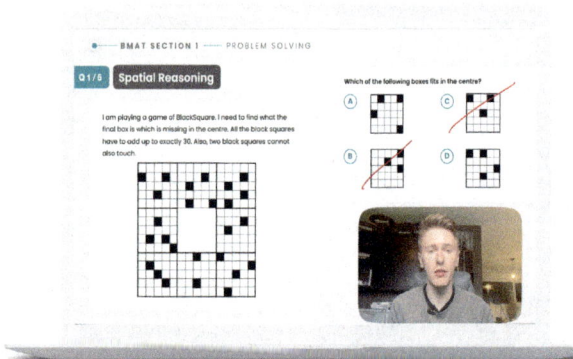

Access our 100+ Tutorials and Materials

Students can put everything they've learned on our UCAT and BMAT Day into practice by completing our self-study UCAT and BMAT practice questions, including worked solutions to guide them through.

Original Question Bank and Videos

We will give your students access to over 10,000 UCAT and BMAT Questions to practise. All the materials come with helpful mini-lectures to guide them through each section and topic.

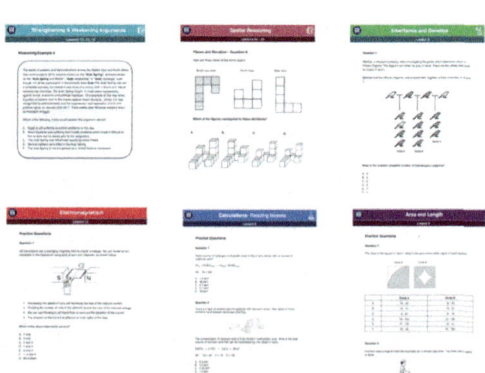

Free Resources!

Alongside the programmes we offer, our medical experts have also written a multitude of free resources to help students study for those all-important exams and interviews.

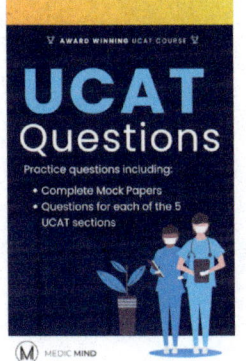

UCAT Practice Questions

With over 5000 free practice questions, our UCAT question banks includes questions and answers organised into the 5 UCAT sections, as well as complete mock papers.

https://www.medicmind.co.uk/ucat-practice-tests/

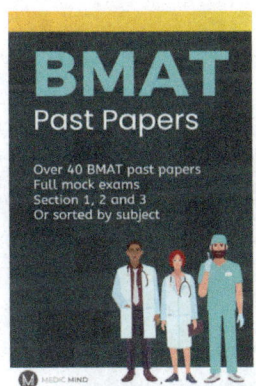

BMAT Past Papers

Your students have access to a vast range of BMAT Past Papers. Search for full mock exams, by section or practise by subject.

https://www.medicmind.co.uk/bmat-past-papers/

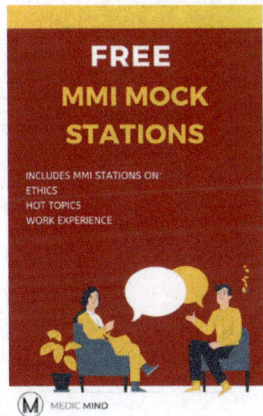

MMI Mock Stations

Free Medicine and Dentistry MMI Scenarios and Questions for you to practise for your MMI Interview. Check out the free MMI Mocks we have for you! https://www.medicmind.co.uk/free-mmi-mock/
https://www.medicmind.co.uk/free-dentistry-mmi-mock/

Free Interview Questions!

Medical-related interviews are not generic and are often tailored to candidate's personal statement, work experience and interests. However, students can prepare and practise answering common interview questions, whether it's independently or under mock conditions. At Medic Mind, we have collated common questions for the medical, veterinary and dentistry interviews to support students in their preparation.

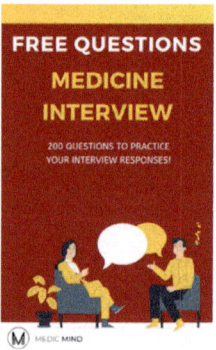

Medical Interview

https://www.medicmind.co.uk/medicine-ucas-guide/medical-school-interview-questions/

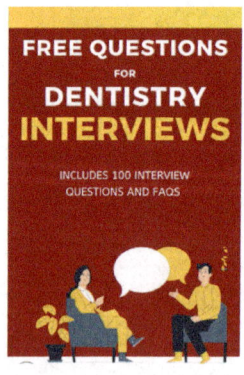

Dentistry Interview

https://www.medicmind.co.uk/medicine-ucas-guide/dentistry-interview-questions/

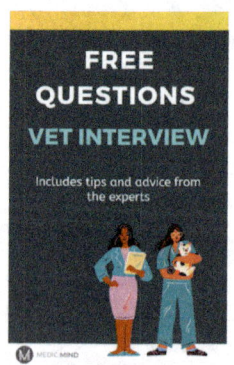

Vet Interview

https://www.medicmind.co.uk/medicine-ucas-guide/top-vet-interview-questions-you-should-be-prepared-to-answer/

What does Medic Mind provide in their Interview Packages?

An engaging and interactive Classroom Day

We will come to your school and provide your students with advice and insight so they can master the biggest hurdle of getting into medical school. We provide university-specific help and online tutorials tailored to you.

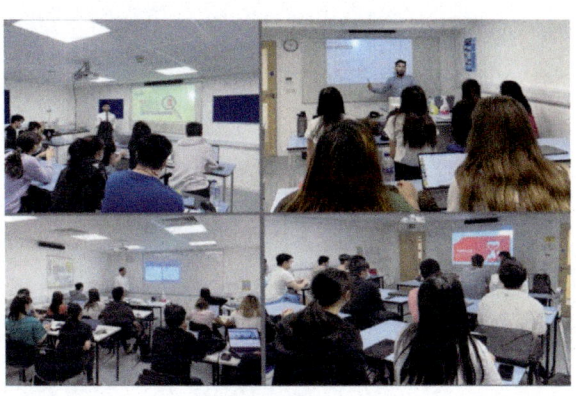

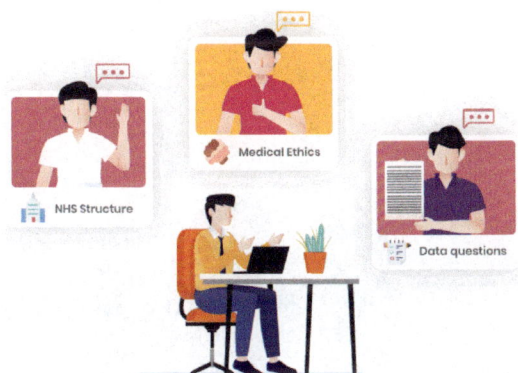

Engaging MMI Circuit, replicating real interviews

Your students will get the opportunity to have a real interview experience by going through a full 20 station MMI Circuit, lasting 2 hours.

Interview Online Course

Your students will receive access to 100+ video tutorials, as well as weekly webinars on a range of topics leading up to the interview.

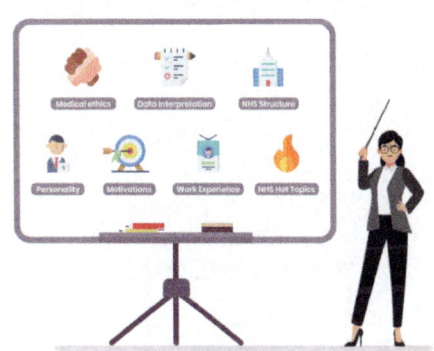

Offered for medicine, dentistry & veterinary interviews.

We look after your students until exam day

Our packages take your students right up to their exam day.

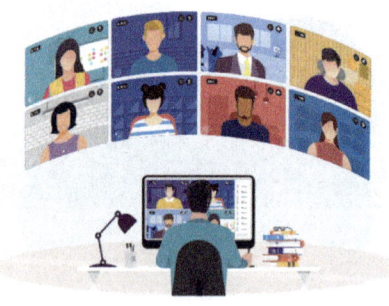

Weekly Webinars

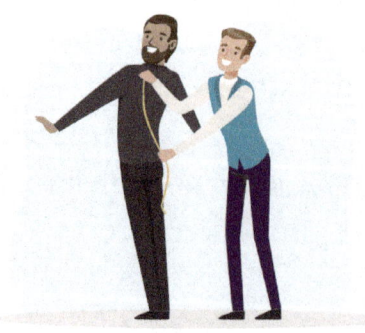

Q&A Support

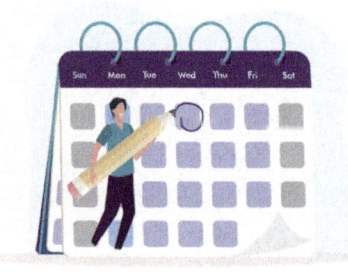

School Revision Planner

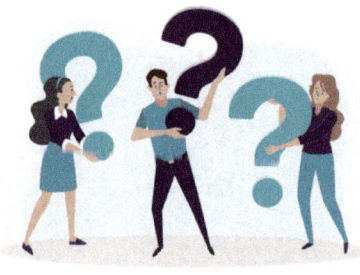

Videos and Question Banks

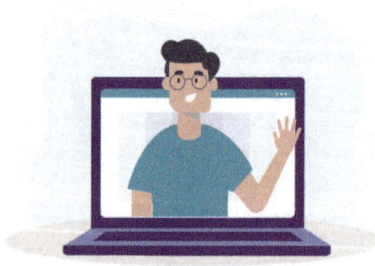

1-1 Tutoring Support

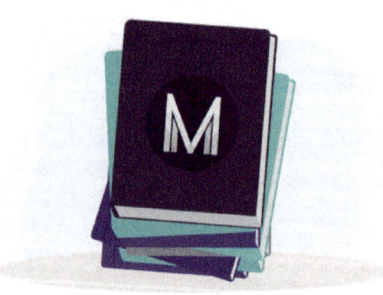

Textbooks & Reading Materials

Live Classroom Day

Our interview courses are fun, engaging and interactive days! Whether it's via an online classroom or in-person, we'll go through the key interview topics whilst providing students the the opportunity to practise, debate and discuss with the teacher!

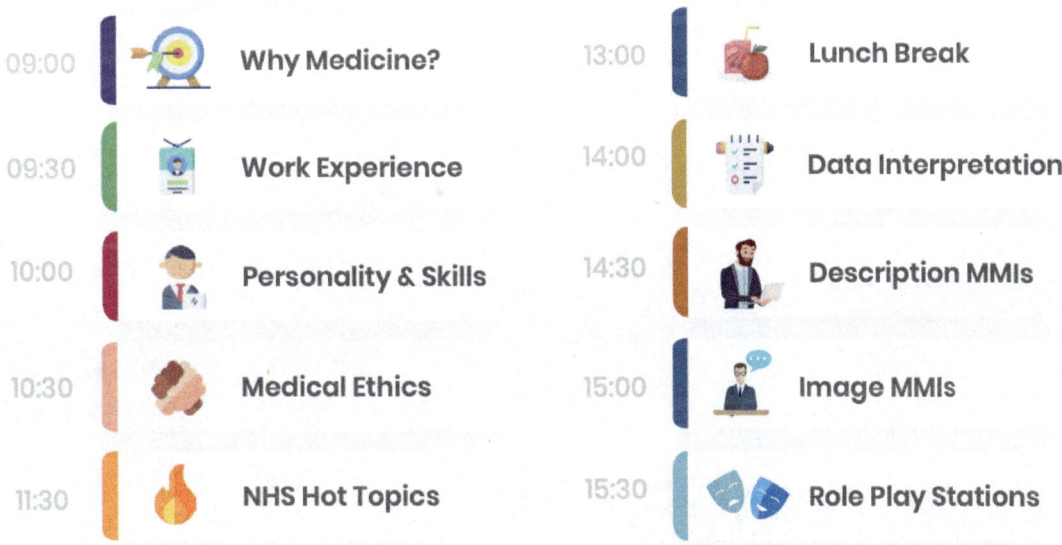

09:00	Why Medicine?
09:30	Work Experience
10:00	Personality & Skills
10:30	Medical Ethics
11:30	NHS Hot Topics
13:00	Lunch Break
14:00	Data Interpretation
14:30	Description MMIs
15:00	Image MMIs
15:30	Role Play Stations

Extra Materials Included:

- ✓ Live Course Day (timetable above)
- ✓ 100 Interview Video Tutorials (via portal)
- ✓ Interview Handbooks for Students
- ✓ 100+ MMI Stations (via portal)
- ✓ Weekly Interview Webinars

Live MMI Circuit

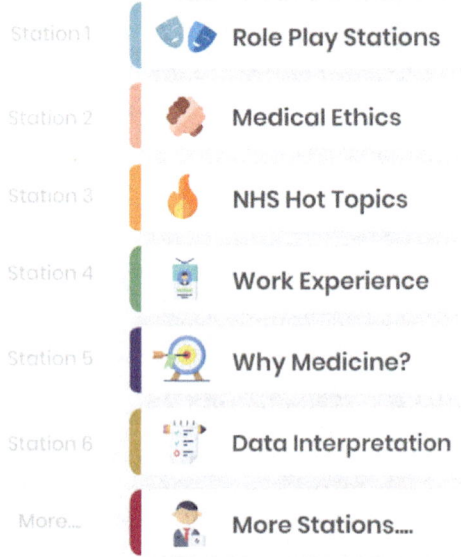

Stations on Key Topics

The MMI circuit will be run via an online classroom. In pairs, students experience 20 stations - they do 10 themselves and they observe their partner doing the other 10, which is a great learning opportunity.

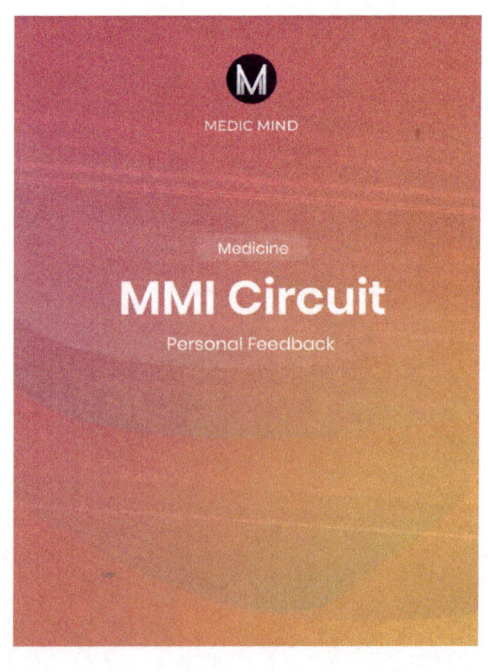

Full Feedback Book

Each student will receive a 70 page feedback document with scores, analysis and examiner insight for each MMI station.

Interview Online Course

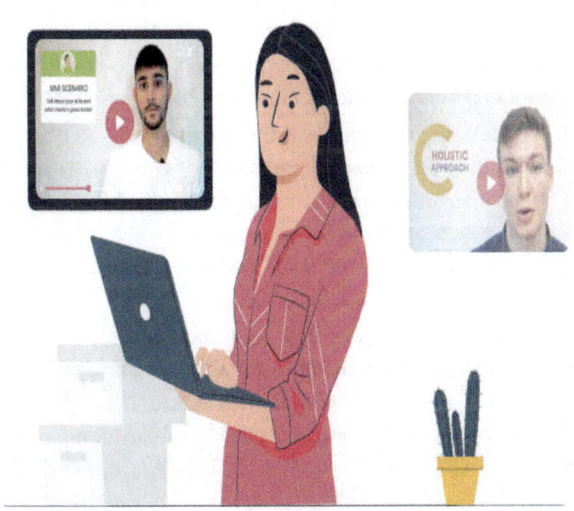

100+ Video Tutorials

Alongside the MMI Circuit Day, you have access to our 100+ online video tutorials and 200+ MMI stations to help you revise all the way until your interview day!

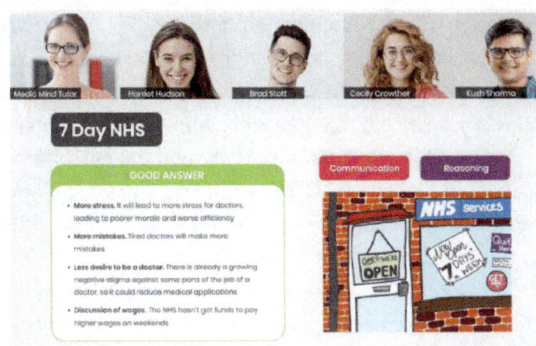

200+ MMI Stations

Your students will have access to a multitude of MMI stations which they can practise in their own time.

Reviews from Students from OIC School Interview Package (2021)

Celia Choi	★★★★★	**It is an extremely helpful day** I found myself enjoying it and feel adequately challenged at the same time. This afternoon gains me an insight into what I really need to answer in face of various types of interview questions. The interviewers at each station are all very nice and helpful in giving really useful and throughout feedbacks to us individually. So far it's been a productive day and I would definitely recommend this to any aspired medics who want to practice a little bit more on interviews to give it a go
Oscar Wong	★★★★	**Can we have more of this please?** This experience was very useful to prepare for interviews, I was exposed to the different questions medical schools may ask, and learnt skills and techniques on how to approach them. I would appreciate it if they ran this perhaps once every month for students. Thanks
Eageon Lai	★★★★★	**Thank you very much!** After the MMIs, the tutors have given very detailed feedbacks on what's good which should be kept, areas of improvements that should be worked on, and solutions guiding us to a better answer. Also, the tutors are very nice and eager to answer our questions in the spare time, on personal statements, applications, entry exams (UCAT/BMAT), tips on MMI interviews, etc.
Karlo Jelic	★★★★★	**Extremely insightful and helpful** This has been an extremely insightful and useful experience. Thank you very much. I have gained a first hand experience on how MMI interviews work which will drastically help me in preparing for the actual interviews. All the interviewers were extremely professional and gave very detailed feedback, which will also help me. The questions were interesting and made me think in a different way, which I really appreciate. Once again, a very useful course which I will definitely recommend to a friend, thank you.
Song Zi Rong	★★★★★	**Really conducive and rewarding** Even though this happened on Sunday afternoon, I could not imagine another more productive way to spend it. I think all interviewers are amazing and these personalised sessions were very helpful in providing individual support. I really enjoy the roleplay MMI, where I had to firmly say "no" for a concert. This was the worst MMI, yet I learned the most from this station. I really reminded me of some tactics which I neglected and I gives an insight on how to properly tackle this problem. I will certainly do better if asked again :))))
Nerd	★★★★★	It was very helpful, and I enjoyed the amount of detailed feedback that was available from having 2 students for 1 tutor. However, there could have been a longer break (maybe 30 mins) considering how the circuit coincided with lunch.

Medical Programmes

Our experienced tutors have all scored in Top 10% and have mastered the application process.

UCAT

- √ Live UCAT Classroom Course, delivered by expert tutors
- √ 8000+ UCAT Questions, on advanced e-learning platform
- √ 100+ UCAT Video Tutorials, accessible from home
- √ UCAT Revision Textbook, with insider tips for the exam
- √ Weekly UCAT Webinars in lead up to the exam

BMAT

- √ Live BMAT Classroom Course, delivered by expert tutors
- √ 1500+ BMAT Questions, on advanced e-learning platform
- √ 100+ UCAT Video Tutorials, accessible from home
- √ BMAT Revision Textbook, with insider tips for the exam
- √ Weekly BMAT Webinars in lead up to the exam

Interview

- √ Live Interview Classroom Course, delivered by expert tutors
- √ Live MMI Circuit, replicating real life interview setting
- √ 100 page Interview Handbook with Practice Questions
- √ 100+ MMI Video Tutorials, accessible from home
- √ Weekly Interview Webinars in lead up to the exam

Vet & Dental Programmes

Our experienced tutors have all scored in Top 10% and have mastered the application process.

UCAT

- √ Live UCAT Classroom Course, delivered by expert tutors
- √ 8000+ UCAT Questions, on advanced e-learning platform
- √ 100+ UCAT Video Tutorials, accessible from home
- √ UCAT Revision Textbook, with insider tips for the exam
- √ Weekly UCAT Webinars in lead up to the exam

Interview

- √ Live Interview Classroom Course, delivered by expert tutors
- √ Live MMI Circuit, replicating real life interview setting
- √ 100 page Interview Handbook with Practice Questions
- √ 100+ MMI Video Tutorials, accessible from home
- √ Weekly Interview Webinars in lead up to the exam

Widening Participation Commitment

Unfortunately, courses like medicine and dentistry, and institutions like Cambridge and Oxford, remain inaccessible for many capable students.

Our mission is to change that.

Through effective, useable and straightforward tutoring and resources, we want everyone to have an equal chance.

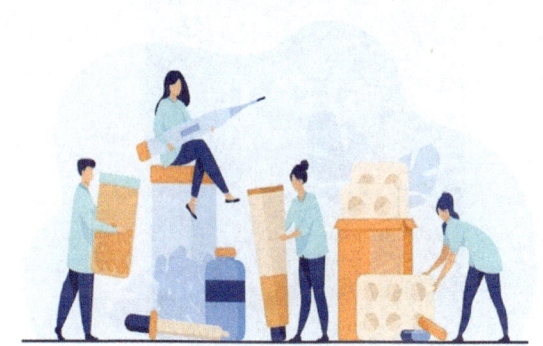

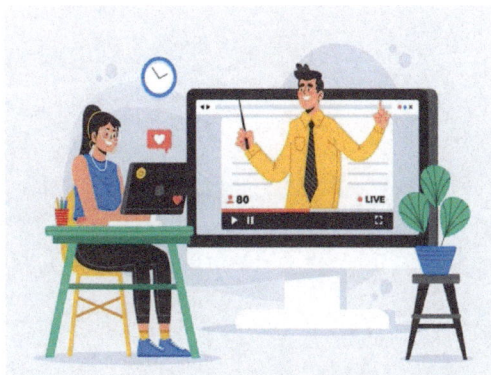

We provide flexible packages that can work in any school context and fit around tight schedules.

You can pick the services that will work best for your students, and students can access our resources from home or school, under our supervision.

Our Use Guarantee means that any service purchased by your school can be used by your students, and recycled between different students and years* as needed.

We don't want costs to be a barrier. Speak to us today and we can cater to your budget and offer bespoke packages.

We have bursaries, discounts and free hours of tutoring available for qualifying schools and students.

Get in touch to find out more!

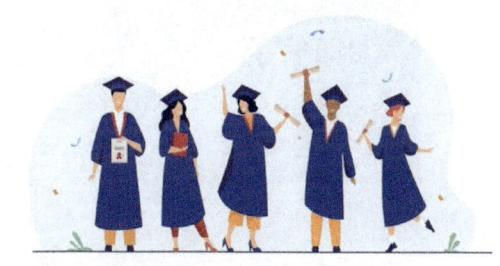

Our Course Textbooks

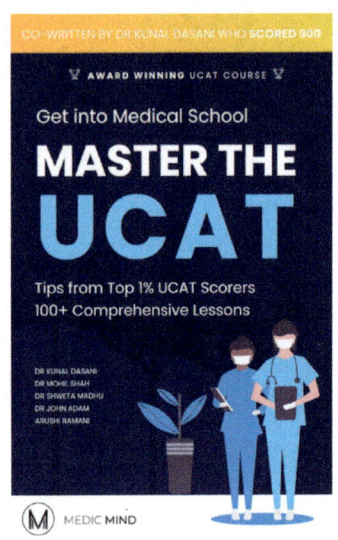

Master the UCAT

With over 100 lessons and insider tips and tricks from UCAT experts and toppers, 'Master the UCAT' includes 100+ lessons with expert tips on timing and efficiency. The book includes new question formats for 2024 and beyond!

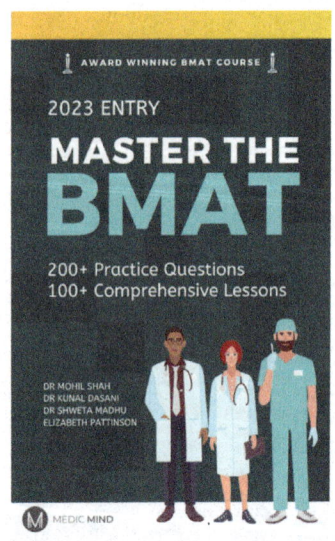

Master the BMAT

With over 200 questions, 100 lessons and insider tips and tricks from BMAT experts and toppers, 'MASTER THE BMAT' is brought to you by Medic Mind, an award-winning company of doctors and medical students.

Our Course Textbooks

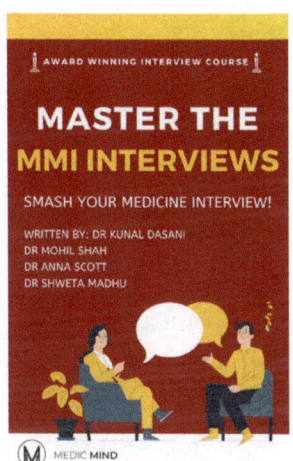

Master the MMI Interviews

This book contains detailed information on topics such as medical ethics, the NHS, motivation for medicine and more. This is the only book available with over 100+ MMI stations with detailed answers. By using this book you'll be able to smash your medicine interview whether it is a panel or MMI.

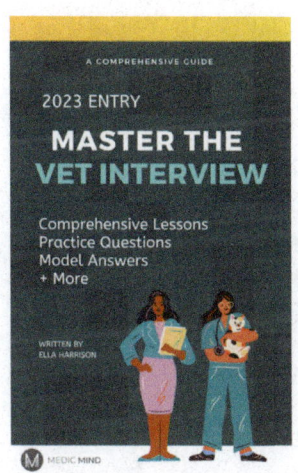

Master the Vet Interview

Filled with top tips and tricks, we will take you through the process step-by-step and tell you everything you need to know, from the different interview formats, types of questions and how to answer them, the selection criteria for every vet school in the UK, key do's and don'ts, and plenty of practice questions for you to use in your preparation.

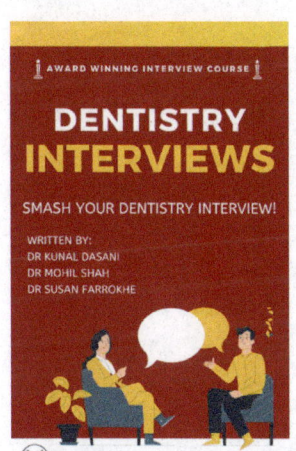

Dentistry Interviews

Applying to dentistry can be tough! The course is super competitive, there's only one shot at your exams and in your interview. 'Dentistry Interviews' includes expert advice, common pitfalls, timing tips, over 120 example questions with answer feedback and NHS hot topics.

Medic Mind UCAS Guide

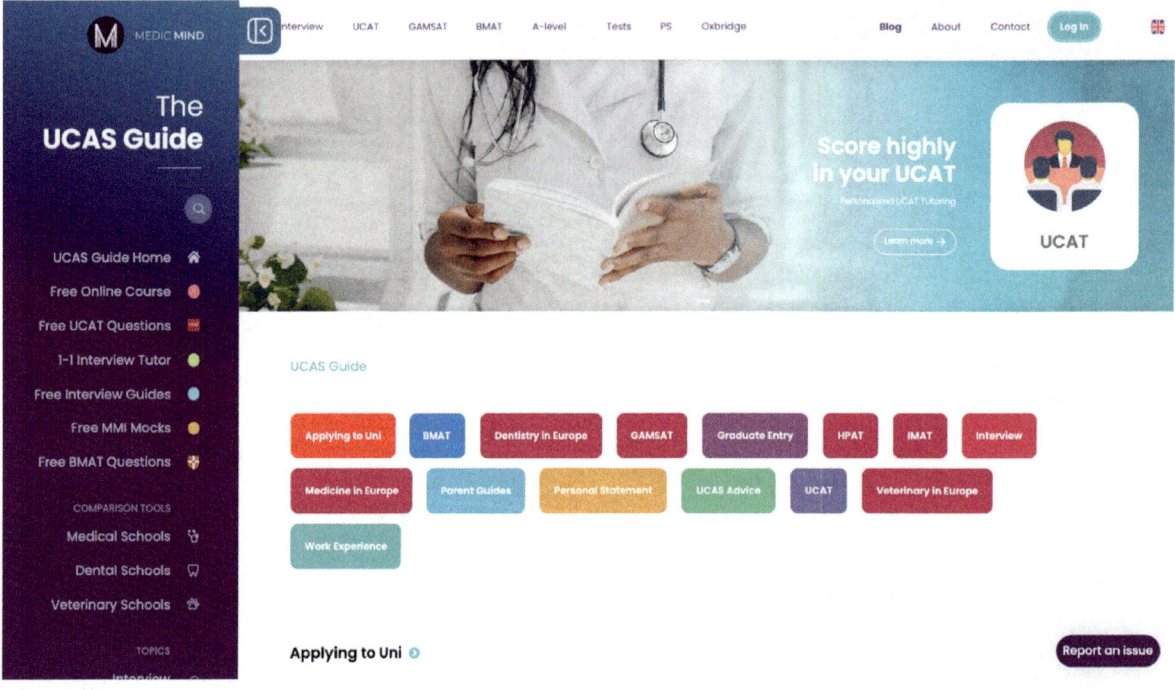

With our Medic Mind UCAS Guide, both you and your students have access to a multitude of articles including the UCAS application process, writing a personal statement and information on admissions assessments.

There is even a teacher's guide with articles explaining the two medical admissions tests in the UK; the UCAT and the BMAT.

With content being updated and added weekly, stay informed with changes, advice and tips!

https://www.medicmind.co.uk/medicine-ucas-guide/

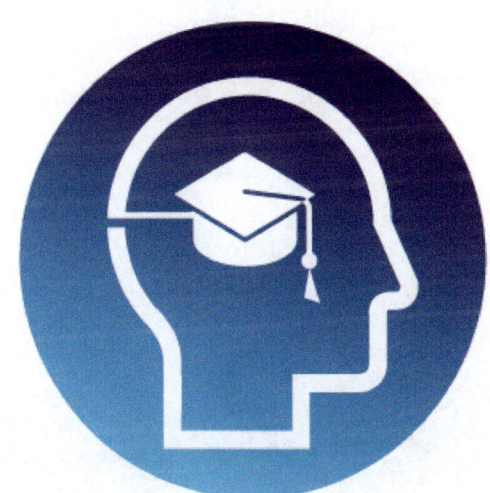

OXBRIDGE MIND

Kieran
Successful Economics Applicant

"I was impressed with the level of support. From the start, I had advice on college choice, the personal statement and preparing for exams. The final hurdle was the interview, and this is what I was most nervous for! My tutor worked through some practice questions and helped me get to the bottom of my nerves."

Your students will receive...

Students will receive the following benefits as part of our Oxbridge Mind programme. In addition to exam support, we can provide help for personal statements, application planning and interviews.

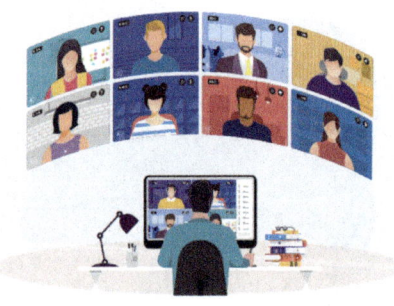

Live Classroom Days

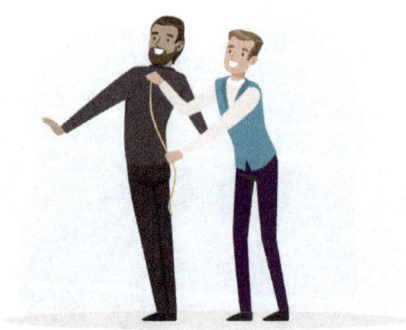

Oxbridge Mentors

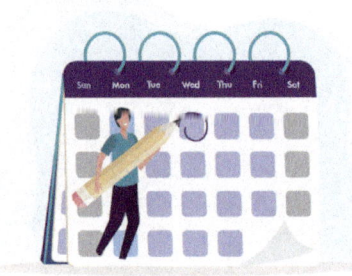

Group Enrichment Seminars

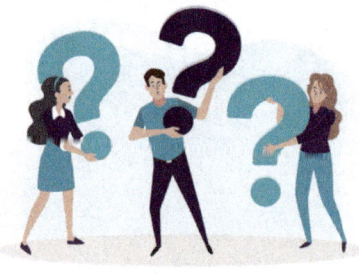

Videos and Question Banks

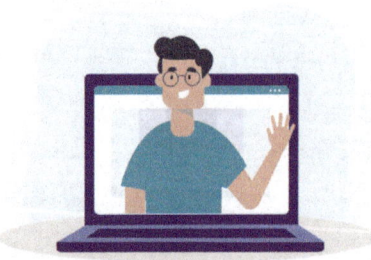

1-1 Tutoring Support

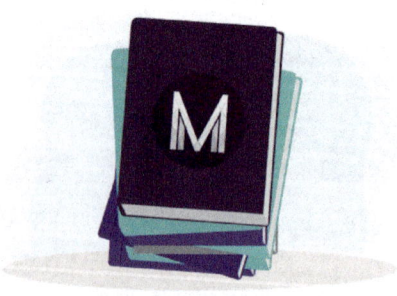

Past Paper Solutions

How can mentoring help you achieve an Oxbridge offer?

1.
Award-winning Strategies

We teach students how to tackle Oxbridge exam questions and improve their understanding of what to expect in the exam.

2.
Essay Planning & Technique

We help students with planning out essay submissions for their application and choosing the work that represents them best.

3.
Video Tutorials & Question Banks

Access to study portals with video tutorials and questions means students can take lead in their own learning.

4.
Enrichment Seminars

These seminars tackle everything from exam preparation, to wider reading and course insights to help students prepare for Oxbridge.

5.
Application Mentoring

We provide experienced Oxbridge help in formulating an application that will get students noticed.

6.
Supportive Oxbridge Mentors

Whether applying as groups or an individual, students will get help from tutors who have been through this themselves!

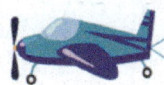 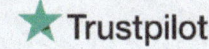 

Free Oxbridge Mind Resources!

Alongside the programmes we offer, our Oxbridge experts have also compiled a multitude of free resources to help students study for those all-important Oxbridge admissions tests. Find them all on https://oxbridgemind.co.uk/past-papers/

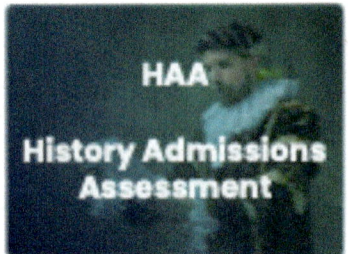
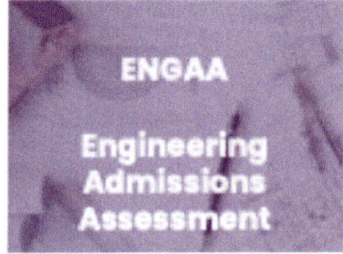
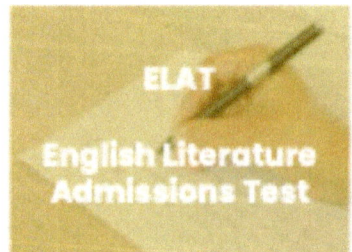
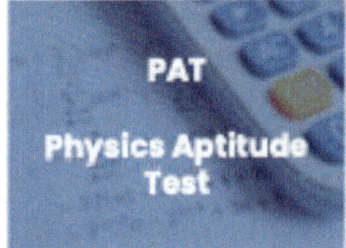
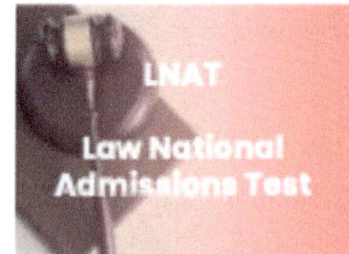
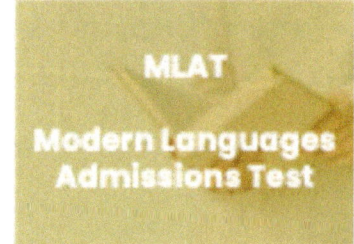
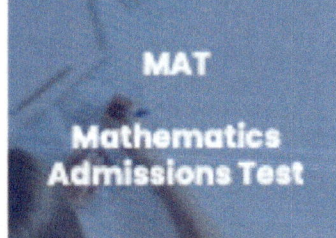
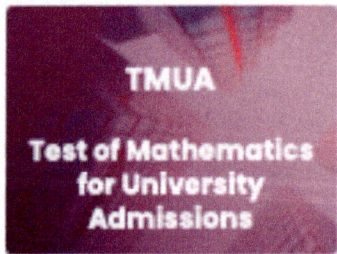
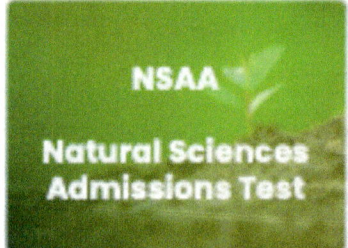
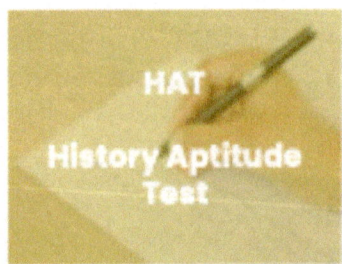
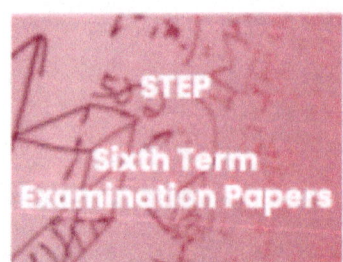
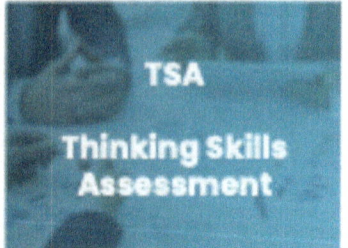

Oxbridge Programmes

Similar schemes available for all Oxbridge Courses -
https://oxbridgemind.co.uk/our-programmes/

Group
- ✓ Classroom Course
- ✓ Question Bank
- ✓ Video Tutorials
- ✓ Past Paper Solutions
- ✓ Essay Plans
- ✓ Enrichment Seminars

Bronze
- ✓ 5 hours 1-1 tutoring
- ✓ 1-1 Application Consulting
- ✓ Classroom Course
- ✓ Question Bank
- ✓ Video Tutorials
- ✓ Past Paper Solutions
- ✓ Essay Plans
- ✓ Enrichment Seminars

Silver
- ✓ 10 hours 1-1 tutoring
- ✓ 1-1 Application Consulting
- ✓ Classroom Course
- ✓ Question Bank
- ✓ Video Tutorials
- ✓ Past Paper Solutions
- ✓ Essay Plans
- ✓ Enrichment Seminars

Gold
- ✓ 20 hours 1-1 tutoring
- ✓ 1-1 Application Consulting
- ✓ Classroom Course
- ✓ Question Bank
- ✓ Video Tutorials
- ✓ Past Paper Solutions
- ✓ Essay Plans
- ✓ Enrichment Seminars

Platinum
- ✓ 30 hours 1-1 tutoring
- ✓ 1-1 Application Consulting
- ✓ Classroom Course
- ✓ Question Bank
- ✓ Video Tutorials
- ✓ Past Paper Solutions
- ✓ Essay Plans
- ✓ Enrichment Seminars

Inside Our Oxbridge Courses...

Video Tutorials

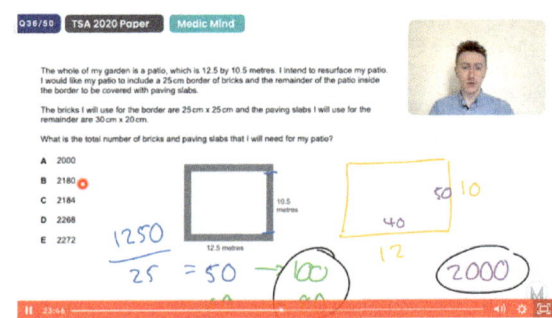

Question Bank

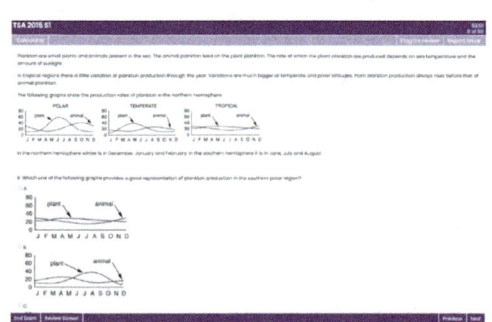

1-1 or Group Webinars

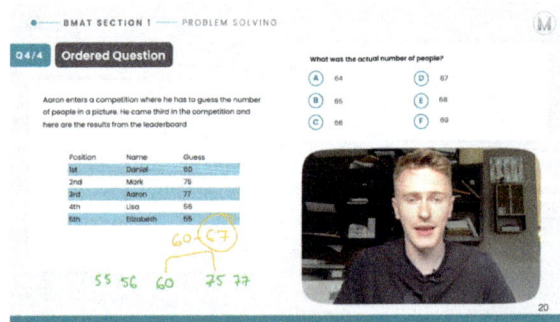

Essay Plans

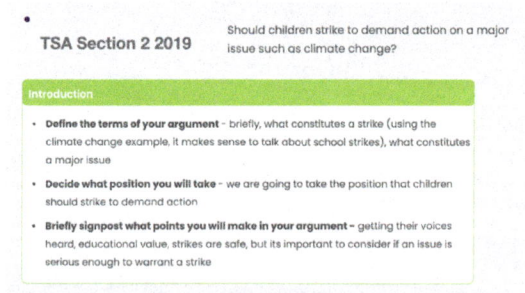

Our Course Textbooks

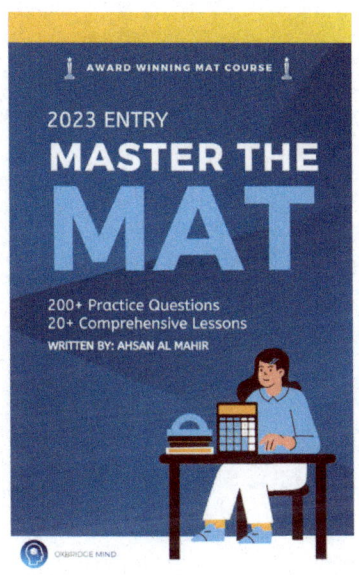

Master the MAT

Are you sitting the Maths Aptitude Test? The MAT is one of the hardest admissions exams and many students often struggle to do well. In this book, you'll grasp all the techniques needed to master the MAT and get into your dream university.

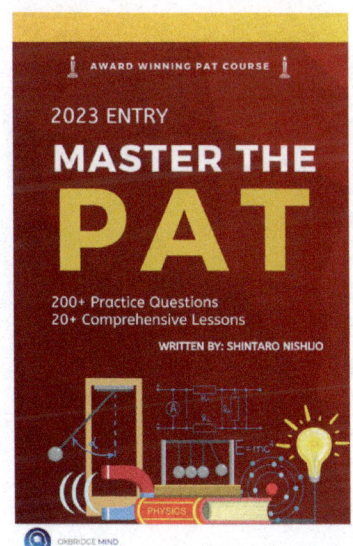

Master the PAT

This book is aimed to prepare students for the Physics Aptitude Test (PAT), which is required for studying Physics at Oxford. It is separated into a section for Mathematics and a section for Physics. There are 200+ practice questions with detailed explanations for every subtopic. With expert tips on timing and efficiency, this book provides you with all the tools necessary to solve any question in the PAT.

Our Course Textbooks

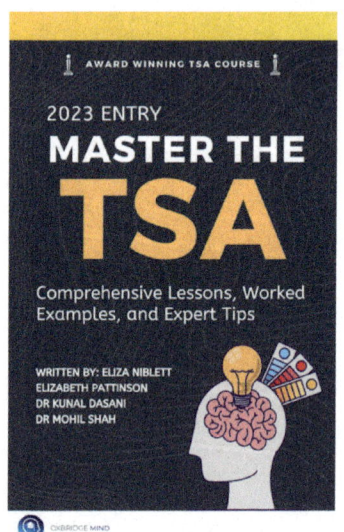

Master the TSA

If you are taking the Thinking Skills Assessment (TSA) for Oxford admissions, this book contains everything you need to know to maximise your success in the exam. Covering both Section 1 and Section 2, it includes worked example questions, lessons and example essays, and expert tips on timing and efficiency. This book will be your guide through the TSA preparation process.

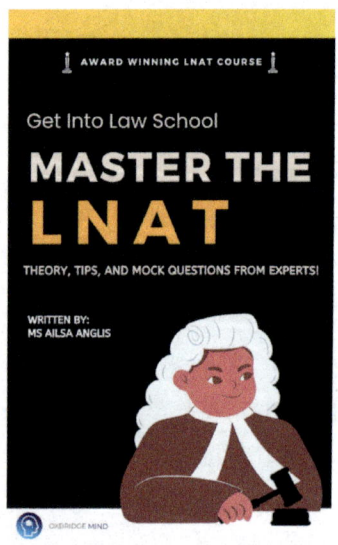

Master the LNAT

With over 30 worked Section A solutions, Section B essay plans and tips and tricks from an LNAT expert, 'MASTER THE LNAT" is brought to you by Oxbridge Mind. This book does not just tell you what the answers are, but why each answer is or is not correct, helping you build the skills you need. The expert tips on the 'perfect' essay formula, timing and efficiency are the perfect complement to the worked solutions, question types and example answers.

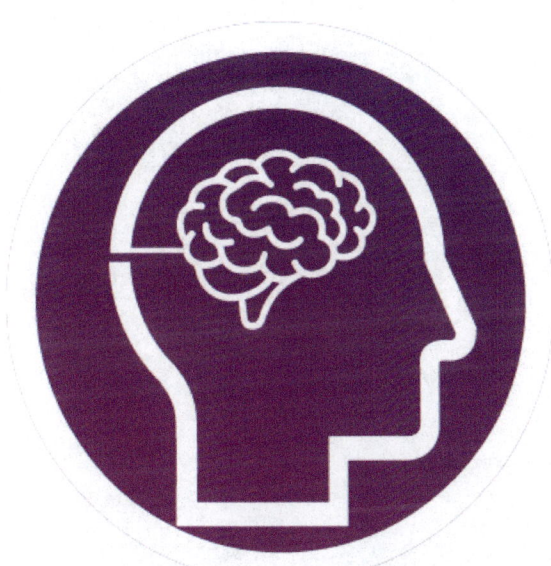

STUDY MIND

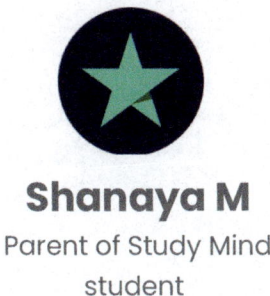

Shanaya M
Parent of Study Mind student

"Brilliant tutors and generally just a great experience! Special thanks to Maya, Julia and Greg for their fantastic tuition of my daughter. I like how the team go the extra mile with their prompt communication and progress

Your students will receive...

Students will receive the following benefits as part of our Study Mind programme. We offer exam support for 11+, GCSEs, A-Levels and IB programmes.

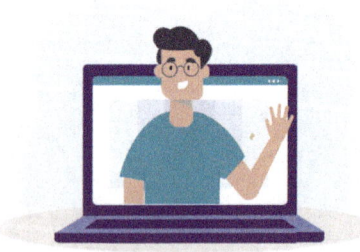

1-1 Tutoring Support

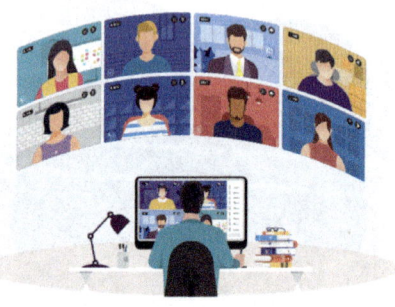

Live Webinar Series

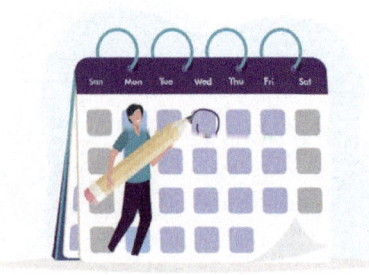

Personalised Study Plans

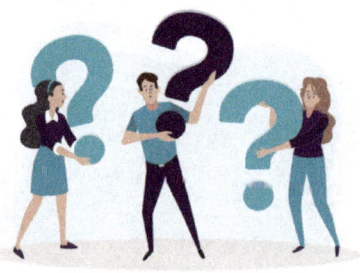

Online Courses and Question Banks

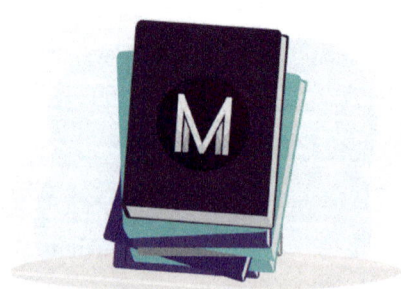

Past Paper Solutions

Study Mind Programmes

Group
- ✓ Classroom Course
- ✓ Question Bank
- ✓ Video Tutorials
- ✓ Past Paper Solutions
- ✓ Essay Plans
- ✓ Enrichment Seminars

Bronze
- ✓ 5 hours 1-1 tutoring
- ✓ 1-1 Application Consulting
- ✓ Classroom Course
- ✓ Question Bank
- ✓ Video Tutorials
- ✓ Past Paper Solutions
- ✓ Essay Plans
- ✓ Enrichment Seminars

Silver
- ✓ 10 hours 1-1 tutoring
- ✓ 1-1 Application Consulting
- ✓ Classroom Course
- ✓ Question Bank
- ✓ Video Tutorials
- ✓ Past Paper Solutions
- ✓ Essay Plans
- ✓ Enrichment Seminars

Gold
- ✓ 20 hours 1-1 tutoring
- ✓ 1-1 Application Consulting
- ✓ Classroom Course
- ✓ Question Bank
- ✓ Video Tutorials
- ✓ Past Paper Solutions
- ✓ Essay Plans
- ✓ Enrichment Seminars

Platinum
- ✓ 30 hours 1-1 tutoring
- ✓ 1-1 Application Consulting
- ✓ Classroom Course
- ✓ Question Bank
- ✓ Video Tutorials
- ✓ Past Paper Solutions
- ✓ Essay Plans
- ✓ Enrichment Seminars

National Tutoring Programme

The National Tutoring Programme (NTP) is a government subsidy which allows you to target tuition for students whose education has been disrupted. You can **subsidise tuition by 60%.**

Study Mind is an approved NTP Partner who work with hundreds of schools to provide online tuition for KS1-KS4 including for SEN.

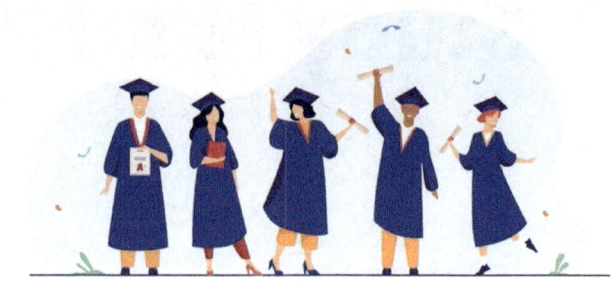

Safeguarding is at the heart of Study Mind. All our tuition takes place online in our secure virtual classrooms. All tutors are vetted and have an enhanced DBS.

We ensure we monitor the quality of our tutoring by providing

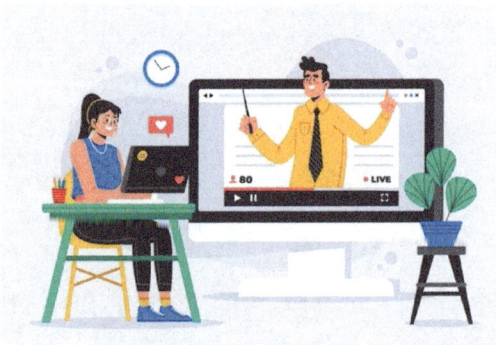

1. Weekly pupil attendance reports
2. Tutor feedback after each tuition session
3. Teacher feedback after each tuition session
4. Your own NTP manager for support
5. Pupil progress measurement after 5, 10 and 15 hours of tuition support

NTP covers 60% of the cost of tuition up to £162 per pupil (£10.80 per hour for 15 hours). The remaining 40% is covered by schools, commonly through their Pupil Premium Fund.

Most schools book a block of 15 hours per student. This allows you to use the lessons throughout the term and make full use of the £162 per pupil.

We know your school has its own needs based on your budget and financial situation. Book a 15-minute call with our NTP Manager to guide you on the best course of action – We can get you up and running within 2 weeks..

Trusted by Schools & Organisations

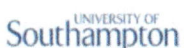 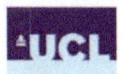 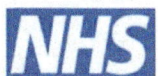 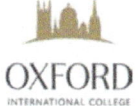

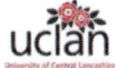 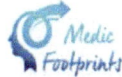 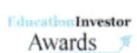 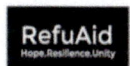 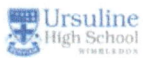

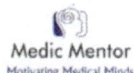 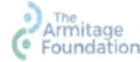 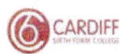 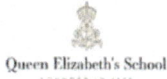 

Ranked as TrustPilot's Top 4 Rated Tutors in the UK

Words from Happy Teachers

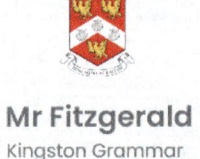

Mr Fitzgerald
Kingston Grammar

I would recommend Study Mind as a reliable organisation to prepare Lower Sixth students for the demands of medical school entrance tests. We will be asking Study Mind back in the Autumn Term to do some Oxbridge training and Interview later in the year.

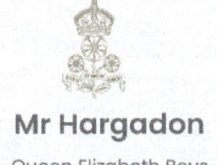

Mr Hargadon
Queen Elizabeth Boys

Study Mind offered a thoroughly professional course which was highly valued by students on the day. The tutor went out of his way to be helpful way beyond the main course and this was most appreciated. I'd recommend Study Mind.

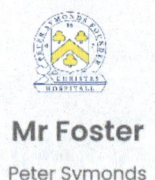

Mr Foster
Peter Symonds

Study Mind enter a very crowded market of providers seemingly offering students a 'golden ticket' to get into university . However, their approach is much more up-to-date, well-informed and is supported by copious notes & activities.

Mrs Bendle
Cardiff 6th Form

Our students and myself were extremely impressed at their professionalism and high quality materials. Their teaching was refreshing, full of engaging anecdotes about their own experiences of being a medical student.

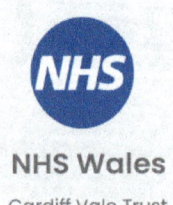

NHS Wales
Cardiff Vale Trust

We were delighted to have Medic Mind in to teach a large group of students in preparation for the UCAT. They provided a structured, engaging session, which was thoroughly enjoyed by the students. Additionally, we were impressed by the wealth of online materials provided to students after the course.

Let's get started!

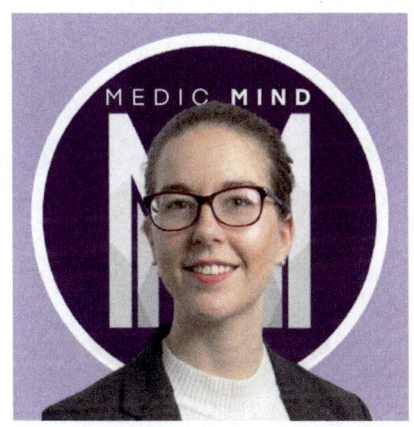

"I'm Daniela, the Partnerships Manager. It's my job to help you to understand what services we offer, how they can be used most effectively in your school, and arrange the packages for you.

We are focused on student success as much as you are, so we are always looking for new ways to help out schools!"

Step 1: Book in your consultation.

There are lots of ways you can arrange a consultation at a time that suits you.

- Book in a direct meeting with me via Calendly https://calendly.com/danielastudymind
- Book in a phone consultation by calling us on +44 20 3305 9593.
- Email us at schools@studymind.co.uk.

During the consultation, we will go through your school, students and the services you are interested in. Feel free to bring in questions!

Step 2: Receive your bespoke package quote.

We will send you a quote based on your needs and budgets as discussed. You can add in additional services at any time. Our Use and Satisfaction Guarantees mean you know that you know the packages will be used and enjoyed in full by your students!

Step 3: Get started!

Our reliable monitoring services mean that we can update you on student progress throughout the time they are studying. We can also arrange feedback for parents and other faculty as required.

Sample Course Materials

The following pages are samples of our upcoming and current course materials that will support students through exam revision and university application process.

A Level Biology Textbook
In the final design stages, this revision book takes students through all AQA specifications and includes top tips and revision ideas.

A Level and GCSE Flashcards
Also in the final design stages, these flashcards will be available for A Level Biology, A Level Chemistry and GCSE Physics. With questions and answers, these flashcards are the perfect accompaniment to any study plan.

A Level Study Buddies
Our revision guides aim to support students in their revision by providing them with summaries of exam topics and what concepts would be helpful to know.

Dentistry Interview Questions
All of our interview courses provide students with example interview questions so they can practice with a Medic Mind tutor, at home or with a friend.

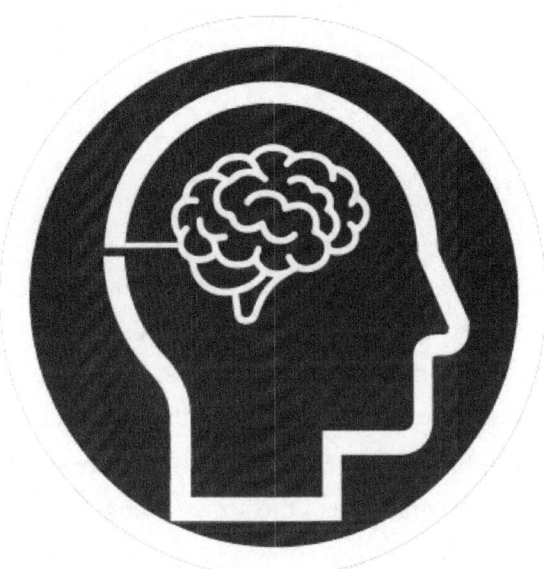

A Level Biology Revision Textbook

COMING SOON!

This is a working sample

Copyright © 2022 by Medic Mind Ltd
All rights reserved. No part of this publication may be reproduced, stored or transmitted in any form or by any means, electronic, mechanical, photocopying, recording, scanning, or otherwise without written permission from the publisher. It is illegal to copy this book, post it to a website, or distribute it by any other means without permission.

This chapter covers the AQA Specification ____

3.1.1 Biological Molecules

Biological Molecules

• Key Aims

1. Characteristics of Biological Molecules.
2. Monomers and Polymers.

• Biological molecules are the building blocks of biology. Biological molecules is a term that is typically used to characterise most molecules and ions in living organisms that contribute to various biological processes (e.g. metabolism, cell division, etc).

• Most biological molecules are organic compounds. Meaning that they are mostly made up of the atom carbon.

• Biological molecules consist of many elements. In addition to carbon, these molecules also consist of oxygen, nitrogen, and hydrogen, which along with carbon makeup 96% of the human body's mass!

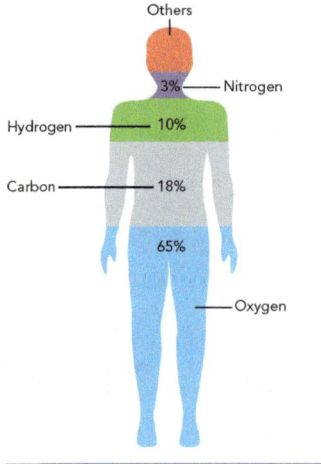

Element	Symbol	Percentage in Body
Oxygen	O	65.0
Carbon	V	18.5
Hydrogen	H	9.5
Nitrogen	N	3.2
Calcium	Ca	1.5
Potassium	P	1.0
Phosphorus	K	0.4
Sulfur	S	0.3
Sodium	Na	0.2
Chlorine	Cl	0.2
Magnesium	Mg	0.1
Trace elements include boron (B), chromium (Cr), cobalt (Co), copper (Cu), fluorine (F), iodine (I), iron (Fe), manganese (Mn), molybdenum (Mo), selenium (Se), silicon (Si), tin (Sn), vanadium (V), and zinc (Zn).		Less than 1.0

Table 1. Chemical Composition of the Human Body: Elements that make up the human body are listed from most abundant to least abundant relative to their mass percentage in the human body.

• There are four major classes of biological molecules. Although there are thousands of various biological molecules, the four major classes we will concern ourselves with in this chapter are carbohydrates, lipids, proteins, and nucleic acids. Together, these four are the most crucial molecules for sustaining life and are made up of the following elements:

• Carbohydrates - C, H, O

• Lipids - C, H, O

• Proteins - C, H, O, N, S

• Nucleic acids - C, H, O, N, P

Monomers and Polymers

- *Monomers are small units that form larger molecules.* Monosaccharides, amino acids, and nucleotides are key monomers, important in making up some important polymers (see table 2).
- Polymers consist of a chain of monomers. Polymers are simply very large, long, and complex molecules which consist of smaller and simpler monomers strung together in a chain (Fig. 1).

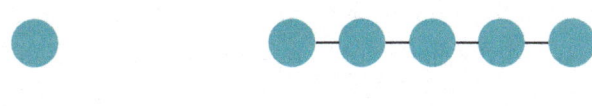

Monomer   Polymer

Fig 1. The Relationship Between a Monomer and a Polymer.

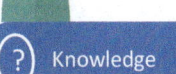

Knowledge

1. What are the four major classes of biological molecules?
2. What monomers and polymers are carbohydrates made from?
3. Are lipids homogenous or heterogenous polymers?

- Polymers can be homogenous or heterogenous. Homogenous means that all of their monomers are the same, and heterogenous means that their monomeric subunits are different. Examples of homogenous polymers are carbohydrates and proteins, and heterogenous polymers include lipids. In later sections of this chapter, we will come across various homogenous and heterogenous polymers.

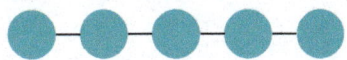

Fig 2. Homogenous Polymer.   Fig 3. Heterogenous Polymer.

- Most biological molecules are polymers. Carbohydrates, lipids, proteins, and nucleic acids are all examples of polymers.

Biological Molecule	Chemical composition	Monomer	Polymer
Carbohydrates	C, H, O	Monosaccharide	Polysaccharide
Proteins	C, H, O, N, S	Amino Acids	Polypeptide
Lipids	C, H, O	Fatty Acid, Glycerol	Lipid
Nucleic Acids	C, H, O, N, P	Nucleotide	Nucleic Acid

Table 2. Monomers and Polymers in Biological Molecules.

This chapter covers the AQA Specification _____

3.1.1 Polymers

Formation of Polymers

- A condensation reaction involves release of water. A condensation reaction is the process by which monomers join together to produce polymers. In the process, there is removal of water (H2O), which enables formation of a covalent bond to link two monomers together.

- A condensation reaction is a synthesis reaction. Synthesis reactions are specific chemical processes by which organic compounds (including biochemical compounds) are made.

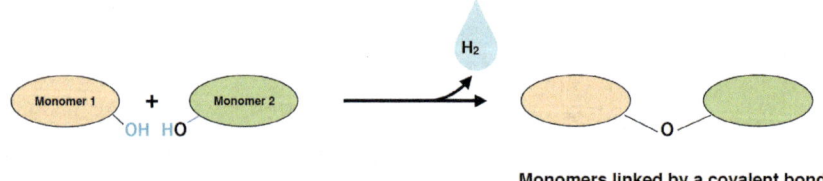

Fig 4. Mechanism of a Condensation Reaction.

Breakdown of Polymers

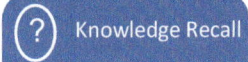 Knowledge Recall

1. What is the process by which monomers join together to form polymers?
2. How can polymers be broken down?
3. In hydrolysis reactions, what does it involve the addition of?

- Polymers put together by a condensation reaction can be broken down by hydrolysis.

- Hydrolysis involves addition of a water molecule. The addition of a water molecule breaks the covalent bond between two monomers (hydro = water, lysis = break down).

- Condensation and hydrolysis are opposite reactions.

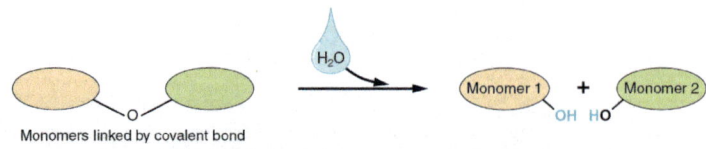

Fig 5. Mechanism of a hydrolysis reaction.

This chapter covers the AQA Specification _____

3.1.2 Carbohydrates: Monosaccharides

Simple and Complex Sugars

- Simple sugars include monosaccharides and disaccharides. Collectively these molecules are referred to as simple sugars.

- Simple sugars can function as small molecules. Monosaccharides and disaccharides can exist on their own and have many important biological roles.

- Simple sugars can also be joined to form complex sugars. Simple sugars can be utilised as monomers to make polymers called complex carbohydrates, which also have various significant biochemical roles.

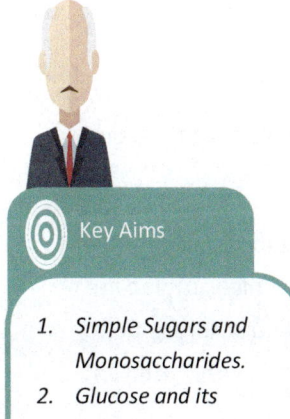

Key Aims

1. Simple Sugars and Monosaccharides.
2. Glucose and its Isomers.

Biological Molecule	Type	Examples
Simple Sugar	Monosaccharide	Glucose, Fructose, Galactose
	Disaccharide	Lactose, Maltose
Complex Sugar	Complex Carbohydrates	Starch, Cellulose

Table 1. Types of sugars.

Monosaccharides

- Monosaccharides are the simplest sugars. Monosaccharides just consist of a single monomer. Examples of monosaccharides are glucose, fructose, and galactose.

- Monosaccharides are organic compounds. This means that they contain the elements C and H, and additionally contain O.

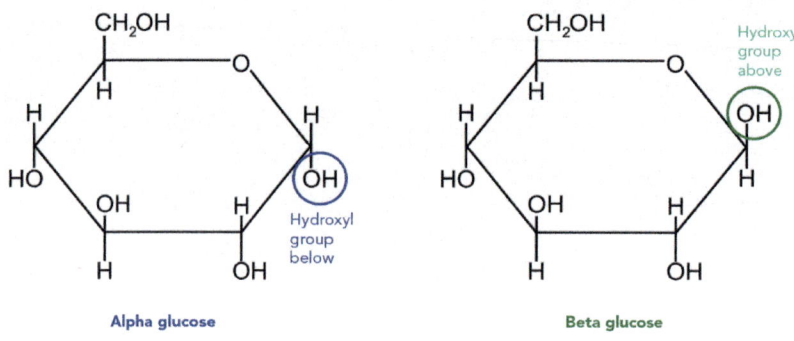

Fig 1. Molecular formulas of α-glucose and β-glucose. Note the structural differences between the two isomers.

Glucose

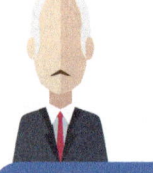

- Glucose is perhaps the most important biological monosaccharide. Glucose is crucial as it is heavily involved in respiration, the process by which living organisms generate energy.

- Glucose is a *hexose sugar*. This means that it consists of 6 carbon atoms.

- Glucose has two key isomers: α-glucose and β-glucose. Memorise their structures for your exam. *Isomers* are chemical molecules that have similar chemical formulas, but different structures due to variation in atom arrangement. Isomers can have very different functions.

In addition to α-glucose and β-glucose, there are other common and biologically relevant monosaccharides, shown in figure 2:

- *Fructose* is commonly found in fruits.
- *Galactose* is a part of the disaccharide lactose that is present in milk.
- *Ribose* is a *pentose sugar*. That means unlike glucose, it only has 5 carbon atoms. It is a common component of genes.

Knowledge Recall

1. Name two types of simple sugars?
2. What is the structural difference between α-glucose and β-glucose?
3. How many carbon atoms are in a glucose molecule?

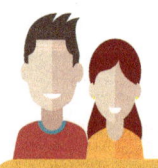

Study Mind Tip

In addition to knowing the structures of α-glucose and β-glucose, it is really important that you spend some time learning the names and structures of some other common and biologically relevant sugars, shown in Figure 2.

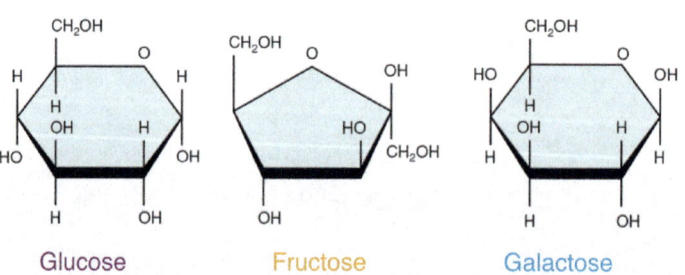

Fig 2. Molecular Formulas of Glucose, Fructose, Galactose, *and Ribose*.

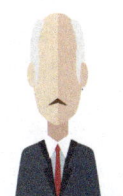

This chapter covers the AQA Specification ____

3.1.2 Carbohydrates: Disaccharides

Key Aims

1. Disaccharides and their Formation.
2. Common Disaccharide Formation Mechanisms

Disaccharides

- Disaccharides are made from two monosaccharides. Disaccharides are dimeric molecules, made of two monomer monosaccharides.

- Disaccharides can be homogenous or heterogenous. The constituent monosaccharides can be the same (homogenous) or different (heterogenous).

- Disaccharides are made via condensation reactions. We learnt about condensation reactions earlier in tutorial 2 Polymers. Disaccharide formation occurs via a condensation reaction between two monosaccharides. Figure 1 below demonstrates this reaction to synthesise the disaccharide maltose.

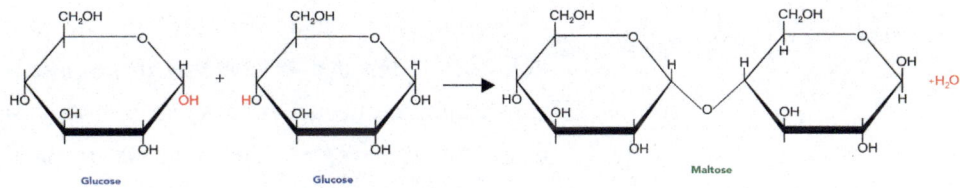

Fig 1. Formation of Maltose. Maltose is formed via condensation between two molecules of α-glucose. The individual glucose molecules are held together by a glycosidic bond (aka glycosidic linkage).

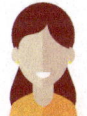

Study Mind Tip

For your exams, you need to know how to draw out the synthesis reactions of some common disaccharides. As such, it is important that you memorise the molecular structures of the common monosaccharides.

- The covalent bond joining two monosaccharides together is a glycosidic bond.

Outlined below for you are the disaccharide forming mechanisms you need to learn:

- Maltose is formed via a condensation reaction between two molecules of α-glucose.

- Sucrose is formed via a condensation reaction between a molecule of glucose and a molecule of fructose.

- Lactose is formed via a condensation reaction between a molecule of glucose and molecule of galactose.

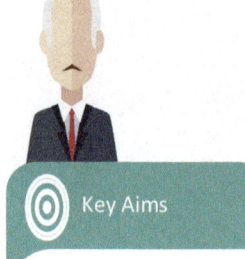

This chapter covers the AQA Specification _____

3.1.2 Polysaccharides

Key Aims

1. Formation and breakdown of polysaccharides..
2. Different types of polysaccharides.

Polysaccharides

- Polysaccharides are complex carbohydrates. Moving onwards from simple sugars (i.e. monosaccharides and disaccharides), we encounter a third class of sugar based compounds which we refer to as polysaccharides.

- Polysaccharides are made by condensation of many glucose units. Polysaccharides are polymers made up of multiple glucose monosaccharides. Like disaccharides, polysaccharides are made through condensation reactions between glucose monosaccharides, resulting in the formation of glycosidic bonds.

- Polysaccharides can be broken down by hydrolysis. Polysaccharides can be broken down into disaccharides or constituent monosaccharides via a hydrolysis reaction This occurs when we test for carbohydrates using Benedict's Test for non-reducing sugars (covered in the later tutorial 20 Testing for Carbohydrates).

There are different types of polysaccharides:

- Glycogen is made from α-glucose. Glycogen is branched and consists of many α-glucose monomers.

- Starch is made from α-glucose. Starch is also made from many α-glucose monomers. There are two types of starch: amylose (non-branched) and amylopectin (branched).

This chapter covers the AQA Specification _____

3.1.2 Function of Polysaccharides

Polysaccharides are involved in various key processes important in the maintenance of homeostasis in an organism.

Starch

- Starch is the key energy store in plants. Most living organisms obtain their energy from glucose. Excess amounts of glucose can be stored in the form of starch, which can later be broken down by a cell to obtain energy.

- Starch is made from amylose and amylopectin. The major starch that we will be concerning ourselves with is a carbohydrate that is actually made up of two polysaccharides of α-glucose: amylose and amylopectin.

- Starch is only found in plants. It is important to note that starches are only found in plants, not animals.

- Starch is insoluble. This is also an adaptation for storage, because starch does not alter the water potential of cells. If it did, there could be an influx of water down an osmotic gradient, making cells swell (and even burst!).

Amylose

- Amylose has a structure adapted for compact storage.

- Amylose is an unbranched chain of α-glucose. Amylose is unbranched, and exists in a coiled helical structure, which gives it an overall cylindrical shape.

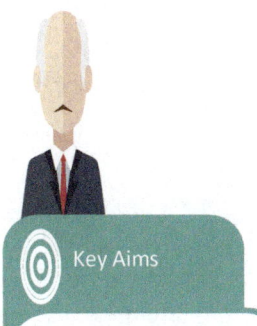

Key Aims

1. Functions of starch.
2. Functions of glycogen.
3. Functions of cellulose.

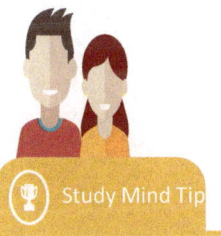

Study Mind Tip

Students often get mixed up between the structure of amylopectin and glycogen. They are both made of branched, α-glucose chains, but glycogen has more branches - a branch per ~10 subunits, compared to per ~20 subunits in amylopectin.

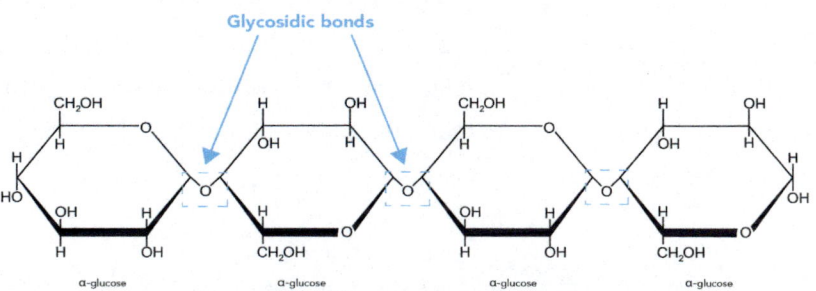

Fig 1. Structure of polysaccharides. This diagram shows an example of a starch polysaccharide called amylose. Notice how it has been formed by joining many α-glucose molecules.

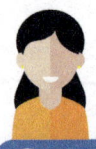

Knowledge Recall

1. Is starch found in both animal and plant cells?
2. Name the two types of starch polysaccharides?
3. What are the structural adaptations of amylase?
4. What are the structural adaptations of amylopectin?

• Amylose is compact and easy to store. The purpose of this structure is simply because it allows the amylose to be neatly compacted, thereby allowing cells to store larger amounts of amylose.

Amylopectin

• Amylopectin has a structure adapted for fast breakdown.

• Amylopectin is a branched chain of α-glucose. Unlike amylose, amylopectin is not in a helical structure, but instead exists as a long chain with branches extending outwards along the backbone.

• Amylopectin is easy to break down. The branched structure means that the glycosidic bonds are much more readily available to various enzymes, which break down these branches in order to release glucose for respiration.

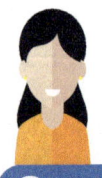

Knowledge Recall

1. Is glycogen found in both plants and humans?
2. Where is glycogen stored?
3. What has more branches, glycogen or amylopectin?
4. What structural adaptation do both starch and glycogen have?

Glycogen

• Glycogen is a key energy store in animals. Whilst starch is the key energy store in plants, glycogen is the key energy store in animals.

• Glycogen also consists of α-glucose. Excess α-glucose molecules can be linked together to form very long polymers of glycogen.

• Glycogen is stored in the liver. Glycogen is typically stored in the liver. When energy levels in an organism run low, signals produced by the hypothalamus in the brain can activate the production of certain endocrine hormones which trigger the release and breakdown of glycogen into glucose. This glucose is then utilised by cells during cellular respiration in order to obtain energy.

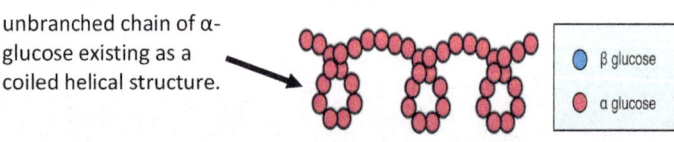

unbranched chain of α-glucose existing as a coiled helical structure.

Fig 1. Amylose.

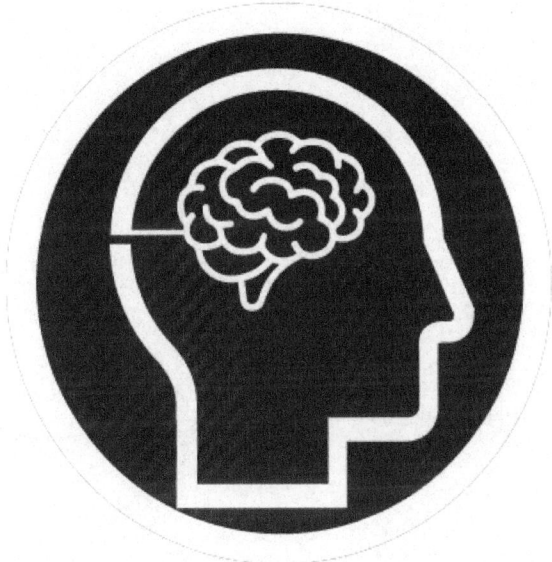

A Level and GCSE Flashcards

COMING SOON!

These are working samples

GCSE Physics Flashcards

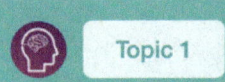 **Topic 1** — **Energy** — 1

Energy cannot be created or destroyed. It can be transferred, dissipated or stored. It is conserved in a closed system. A system is an object or group of objects.

Open systems are able to exchange energy and matter with their surroundings

Closed systems are unable to exchange energy and matter with their surroundings

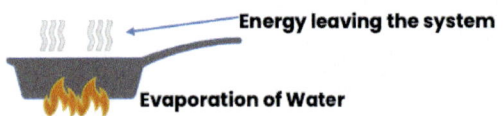
Evaporation of Water — Energy leaving the system

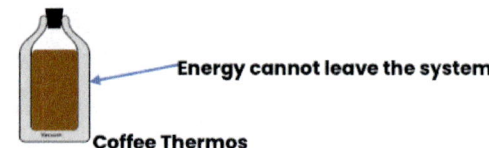
Coffee Thermos — Energy cannot leave the system

When you boil water in a saucepan, heat energy is able to leave the system in the form of steam. As this energy gets transferred, the system is changing.

When you pour coffee into an insulated thermos flask and close the lid, heat energy cannot leave the system. This means you have created a closed system where no energy or matter can be transferred.

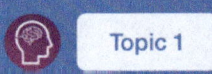 **Topic 1** — **Energy** — 2

What is the difference between an open system and a closed system?
_____
_____
_____

A drinks company proposes a design for a thermos flask. The company have designed the flask so that it keep drinks hot for as long as possible. The diagram shows their design. Describe how each feature of the design will help keep the drink hot.

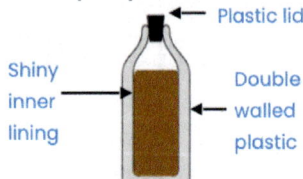
Plastic lid
Shiny inner lining
Double walled plastic

What is the difference between an open system and a closed system?
In an open system, energy can be transferred to the surroundings whereas in a closed system energy cannot leave the system and be transferred.

Describe how each feature of the design will help keep the drink hot.

Plastic lid– poor conductor that will keep heat in. Double walled plastic container – poor conductor. Shiny silver lining – will reflect the heath back to the liquid.

Topic 2 — Energy stores

1. Thermal energy	2. Kinetic energy	3. Chemical energy	4. Magnetic energy
is due to kinetic energy of particles in a system. Example: fire	due to the movement of particles in systems Example: a moving car	Is stored energy in a system Example: batteries	Is due to the attraction between magnetic objects Example: magnets

5. Gravitational potential energy (GPE) — Is due to height above ground. Example: potential energy in a diver

Types of energy stores

6. Elastic potential energy (EPE) — Is stored mechanical energy, often due to the distortion of an object's shape. Example: elastic potential energy in an elastic band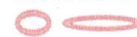

7. Electrostatic energy	8. Nuclear energy	9. Light energy	10. Sound energy
Due to presence of an electric field Example: electrostatically charged clothes	Is due to nuclear fission Example: nuclear power station	Is due to light Example: a lamp	Sound energy is due to sound (vibration of particles) Example: playing music

Topic 2 — Energy stores

Thermal energy	_____	Chemical energy	_____
is due to kinetic energy of particles in a system. Example: _____	is due to the movement of particles in a system Example: a moving car	Is stored energy in a system Example: _____	Is due to the attraction between magnetic objects Example: magnets

_____ — Is due to height above ground. Example: potential energy in a diver

Fill in the missing boxes

Elastic potential energy (EPE) — Is stored mechanical energy, often due to the distortion of an object's shape. Example: _____

Electrostatic energy	Nuclear energy	Light energy	Sound energy
Due to the presence of an electric field Example: _____	Is due to nuclear fission Example: nuclear power station	Is due to light Example: _____	Sound energy is due to sound (vibration of particles) Example: playing music

Kinetic energy

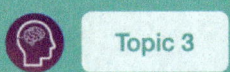
Topic 3

Moving objects having kinetic energy.
Kinetic energy is the energy which a body possesses by virtue of being in motion.
Kinetic energy depends on an object's speed and mass.

If 2 objects have the same speed, the heavier object will have more **kinetic energy.**

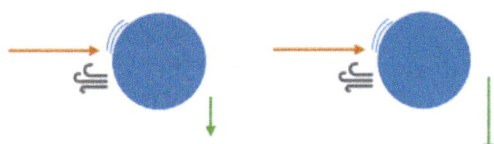

If two objects have the same mass, the faster moving object will have more **kinetic energy**

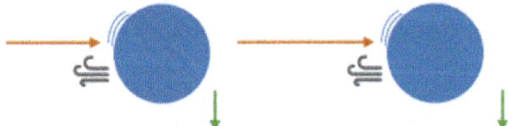

Calculating kinetic energy

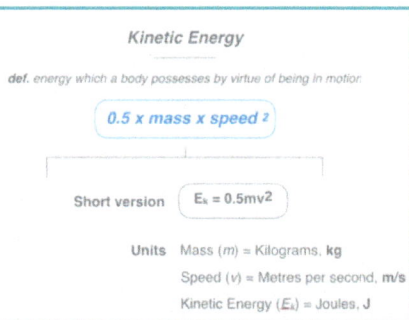

Kinetic Energy

def. energy which a body possesses by virtue of being in motion.

0.5 x mass x speed ^{2}

Short version $E_k = 0.5mv^2$

Units   Mass (m) = Kilograms, **kg**
Speed (v) = Metres per second, **m/s**
Kinetic Energy (E_k) = Joules, **J**

Kinetic energy

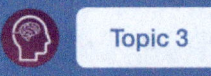
Topic 3

What is kinetic energy? Which two factors affect the kinetic energy of an object?
_____
_____
_____
_____

A runner with a mass of 70kg moves at 5m/s. What is its kinetic energy in kJ?

What is kinetic energy? Which two factors affect the kinetic energy of an object?

Kinetic energy is the energy which a body possesses by virtue of being in motion. Depends on an object's speed and mass.

A runner with a mass of 70kg moves at 5m/s. What is its kinetic energy in kJ?

$E_k = 1/2mv^2$

Kinetic energy = $0.5 \times 70 \times (5)^2$
Kinetic energy = 875 joules

Kinetic energy = 0.875 kJ

Topic 4 — Gravitational potential energy

Gravity is a force that attracts objects towards the centre of the earth.
To overcome gravity and lift an object, work is done which requires energy.
As an object is lifted in the air, it gains gravitational potential energy (GPE).
GPE is the energy stored in an object positioned at a height above or below the surface of the earth.
GPE depends on the object's height and mass

Example:
Gain in GPE = work done in climbing the diving board

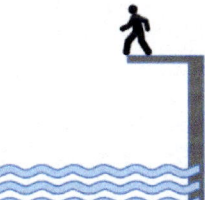

Calculating GPE:

mass x gravitational field strength x height

Short version: $E_p = mgh$

Units:
- Mass (m) = Kilograms, kg
- Gravitational Field Strength (g) = Newtons per kilogram, N/kg
- Height (h) = Metres, m
- Gravitational Potential Energy (E_p) = Joules, J

Topic 4 — Gravitational potential energy

What is gravitational potential energy (GPE) and what two factors affect the GPE of an object?

_____
_____
_____
_____

Sam weighs 75kg and climbs a diving board that is 10m tall. Calculate his GPE in kJ giving your answer to 1 d.p. Take the value of g as 9.8 N/kg.

What is gravitational potential energy (GPE) and what two factors affect the GPE of an object?

GPE is the energy stored in an object positioned at a height above or below the surface of the earth. GPE is dependent on the mass and height of an object.

Sam weighs 75kg and climbs a diving board that is 10m tall. Calculate his GPE in kJ giving your answer to 1 d.p. Take the value of g as 9.8 N/kg

$E_p = mgh$

GPE = 75 x 9.8 x 10
GPE = 7350 J

GPE = 7.4 kJ

A Level Biology Flashcards

AQA 3.1.1 — Polymers

Polymers are chains of monomers. They can be **homogenous** or **heterogenous**. Most biological molecules are polymers (e.g. proteins, lipids)

Polymers are formed during **condensation reactions**

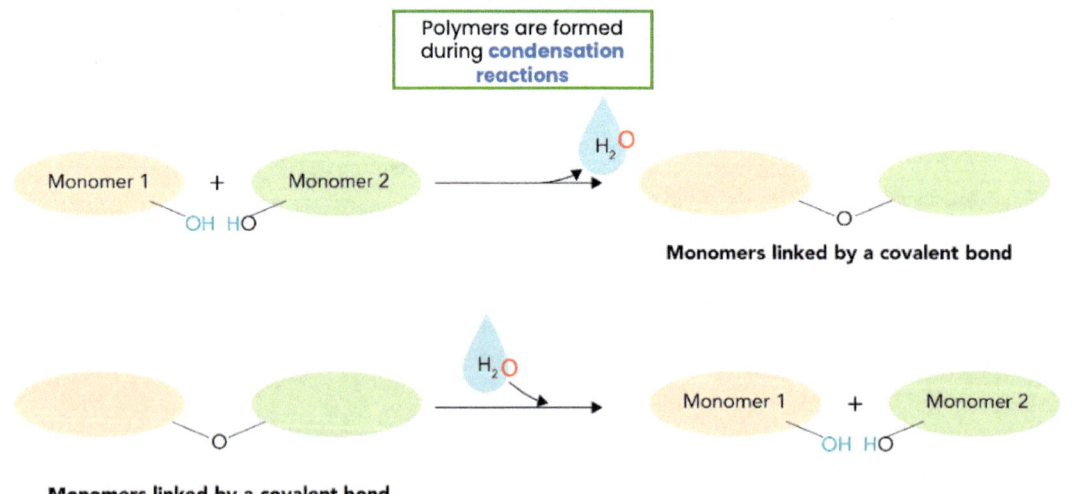

Monomer 1 + Monomer 2 → Monomers linked by a covalent bond (+ H_2O)

Monomers linked by a covalent bond → Monomer 1 + Monomer 2 (+ H_2O)

Polymers are broken down during **hydrolysis reactions**.

AQA 3.1.1 — Polymers

Fill in the missing boxes on this table.

Biological Molecules	Monomer	Polymer
Proteins		Polypeptide
	Fatty Acid, Glycerol	
Nucleic Acids	Nucleotide	

Fill in the missing boxes on this table.

Biological Molecules	Monomer	Polymer
Proteins	Amino Acids	Polypeptide
Lipids	Fatty Acid, Glycerol	Lipid
Nucleic Acids	Nucleotide	Nucleic Acid

Identify what type of bonds are formed/broken in condensation reactions.

_____
_____

Identify what type of bonds are formed in condensation reactions.

Covalent bonds are formed during condensation reactions.

Carbohydrates: Monosaccharides

AQA 3.1.2

Monosaccharides are **organic compounds** containing elements **C, H,** and **O**. They are the simplest sugars which are made of just one monomer.

Here are some examples of monosaccharides:

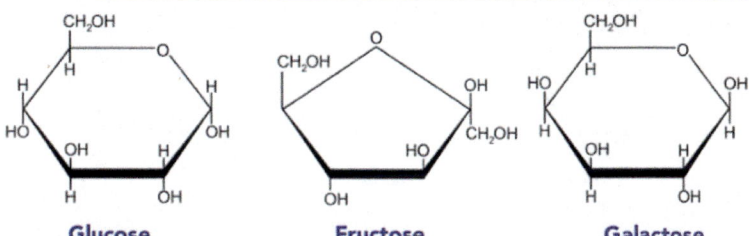

Glucose   **Fructose**   **Galactose**

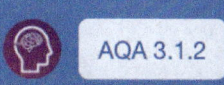

Glucose has two important isomers, α-glucose and β-glucose.

Alpha glucose   **Beta glucose**

Carbohydrates: Monosaccharides

AQA 3.1.2

Define hexose sugar.

_____
_____
_____

Define hexose sugar.

A hexose sugar is a monosaccharide that has 6 carbon atoms.

Explain the structural difference between α-glucose and β-glucose.

_____
_____
_____
_____

Explain the structural difference between α-glucose and β-glucose.

The position of the OH group and H group attached to carbon 1 on α-glucose is opposite to that of β-glucose. This affects which polymer will form from them.

Carbohydrates: Disaccharides

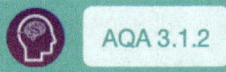

Disaccharides are made from two **monosaccharides**. They are joined together by a **glycosidic bond** between two monosaccharides.

They are formed by **condensation reactions.**

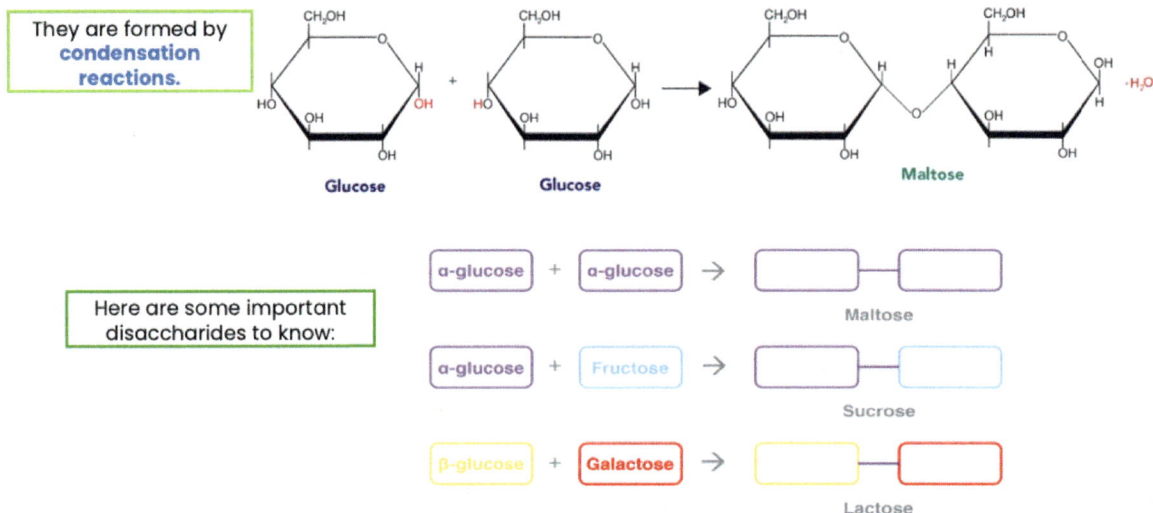

Here are some important disaccharides to know:

α-glucose + α-glucose → Maltose

α-glucose + Fructose → Sucrose

β-glucose + Galactose → Lactose

Carbohydrates: Disaccharides

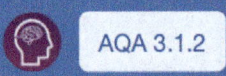

Identify the products of a condensation reaction between two monosaccharides.

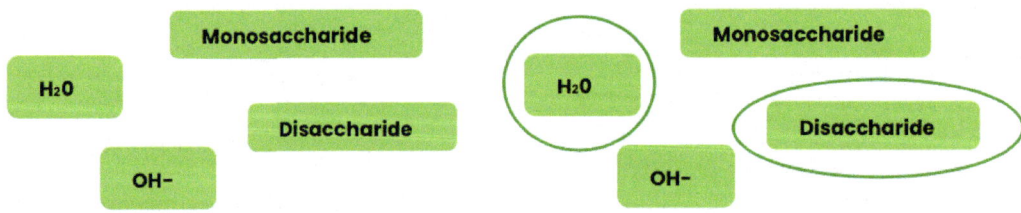

Which isomer of glucose is present in a lactose molecule?

_____

Which isomer of glucose is present in a lactose molecule?

β-glucose

Carbohydrates: Polysaccharides

AQA 3.1.2

Polysaccharides are complex carbohydrates made by condensation of many glucose units.

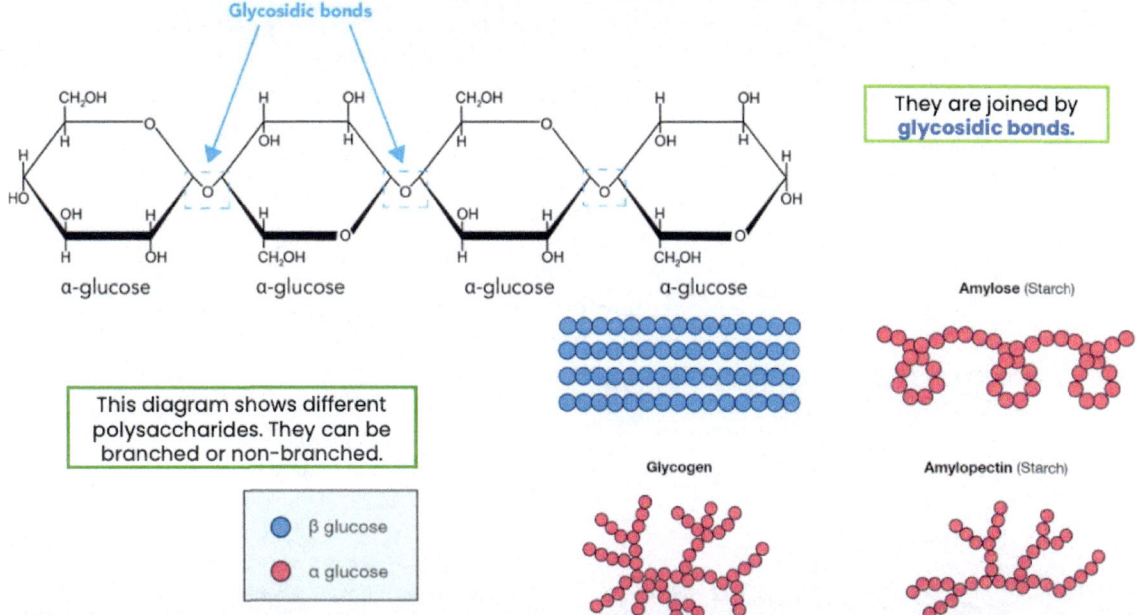

They are joined by glycosidic bonds.

This diagram shows different polysaccharides. They can be branched or non-branched.

- β glucose
- α glucose

Carbohydrates: Polysaccharides

AQA 3.1.2

Describe the similarities and differences between the three major polysaccharides: glycogen, starch, and cellulose.

Describe the similarities and differences between the three major polysaccharides: glycogen, starch, and cellulose.

They are all homogeneous molecules made of glucose. Glycogen and starch are both composed of α-glucose, whereas cellulose is composed of β-glucose. Cellulose and amylose (starch) are non-branched, while glycogen and amylopectin (starch) are branched.

A Level Chemistry Flashcards

AQA 3.1.1.1 Subatomic Particles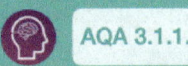

An element is made of one type of atom. **Elements** are made up of atoms, and each element only has one type of atom.

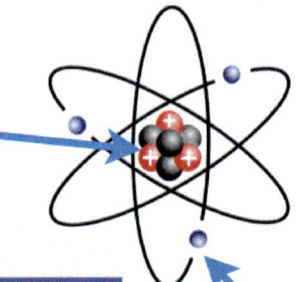
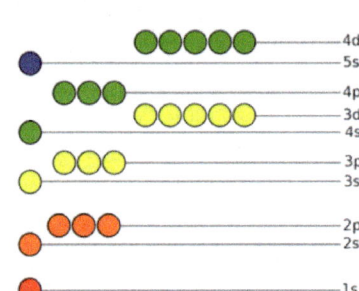

Protons + Neutrons
Atoms are mostly empty space surrounding a very small, dense nucleus that contains both the protons and the neutrons

Electrons
The electrons are found in orbitals which surround the nucleus. Electrons can have different energy levels, and each distance from the nucleus represents a different energy level

Subatomic Particle	Relative Charge	Relative Mass
Proton	1	1
Neutron	0	1
Electron	-1	Negligible (1/2000)

AQA 3.1.1.1 Subatomic Particles

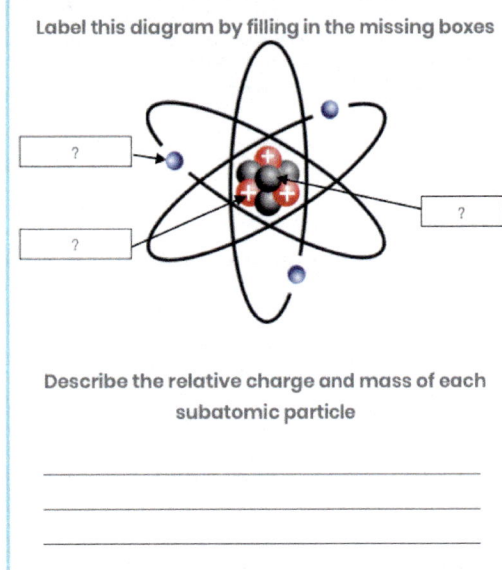

Label this diagram by filling in the missing boxes

Describe the relative charge and mass of each subatomic particle

_____
_____
_____

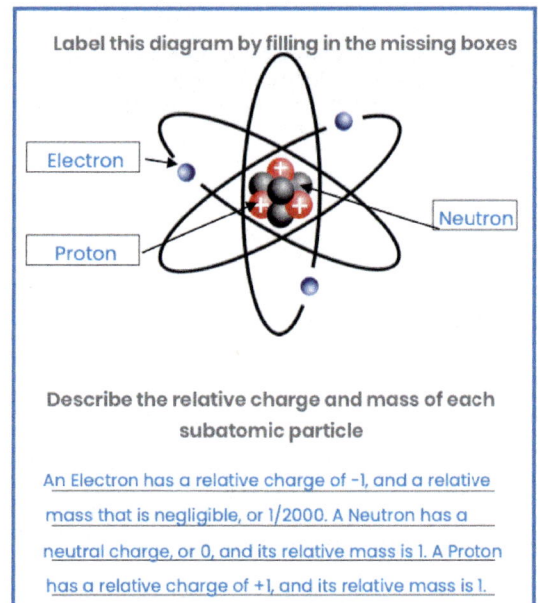

Label this diagram by filling in the missing boxes

Describe the relative charge and mass of each subatomic particle

An Electron has a relative charge of -1, and a relative mass that is negligible, or 1/2000. A Neutron has a neutral charge, or 0, and its relative mass is 1. A Proton has a relative charge of +1, and its relative mass is 1.

Subatomic Particles

AQA 3.1.1.1

Dalton's model of the atom. John Dalton suggested that all matter was composed of tiny, indivisible, **solid spheres** which he called atoms and that different elements where made up of different atoms.

Thompson's model of the atom. In 1897 J.J. Thompson first discovered the **electron**. He suggested that atoms consisted of negatively charged particles embedded in a sea of positive charge, like plums in a pudding, hence the **'plum pudding model'** name.

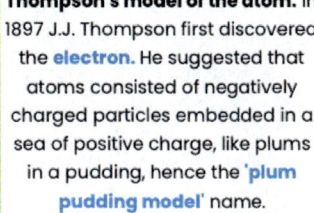

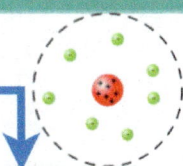

Rutherford's model of the atom. In 1909, Ernest Rutherford conducted an experiment where he fired positively charged **alpha particles** through a thin sheet of gold. Most of the particles passed straight through but a small amount were deflected backwards. He therefore proposed that atoms consisted of a **tiny, dense, positively charged core** or nucleus surrounded by a **cloud of negatively charged electrons**.

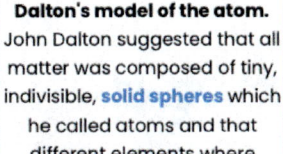

Chadwick's model of the atom. In 1932 Chadwick suggested there must exist another particles in the nucleus along with protons, which would otherwise strongly repel each other. James Chadwick later discovered the **neutron**.

Bohr's model of the atom. In 1920 Niels Bohr proposed that electrons could only exist in **shells or orbits** at **different energy levels** around the nucleus. When electrons moved from from one shell to another, they emitted or absorbed **electromagnetic radiation** of fixed frequency. This model was later refined to include **sub-shells**.

Subatomic Particles

AQA 3.1.1.1

Describe the Rutherford's gold foil experiment, its findings, and its significance. Draw his model.

_____
_____
_____
_____

Describe the Thompson's model of the atom.

_____
_____
_____
_____

Describe the Rutherford's gold foil experiment, its findings, and its significance. Draw his model.

The Rutherford gold foil experiment involved firing +ve alpha particles through a thin gold sheet. Most particles passed straight through the sheet, but some were deflected backwards. Rutherford proposed this was because it hit a very small, dense, positive nucleus.

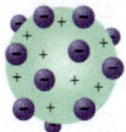

Describe the Thompson's model of the atom.

The Thompson model was the first to include electrons in their model. It consisted of a positively charged atom onto which smaller negatively charged particles were embedded into. This is called the 'plum pudding model'.

Subatomic Particles — AQA 3.1.1.1

The **mass number** is the total number of protons and neutron which are found in the nucleus. Electrons have a negligible mass, so we don't usually count it when working out the mass of an atom.

The **atomic number** is the number of protons in the nucleus. Each element has its own atomic number, characteristic of the element and helping you recognise it.

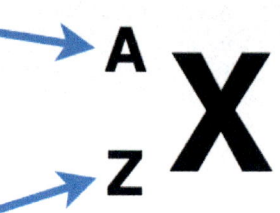

$$^{A}_{Z}X$$

Ions are formed from atoms when electrons are transferred between them

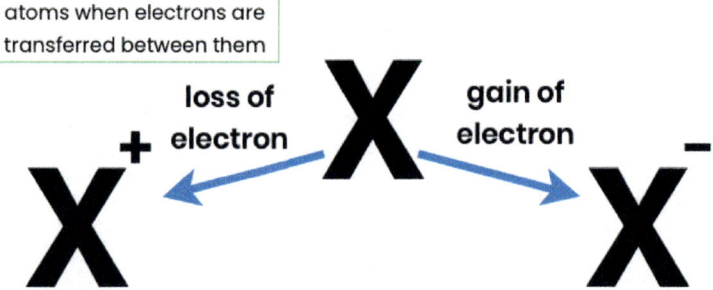

loss of electron → X^+ Cation
gain of electron → X^- Anion

Mass number = protons + neutrons
Atomic number = protons
Number of neutrons = mass number − atomic number
Number of electrons = number of protons (in an atom)

Subatomic Particles — AQA 3.1.1.1

Label this diagram by filling in the missing boxes

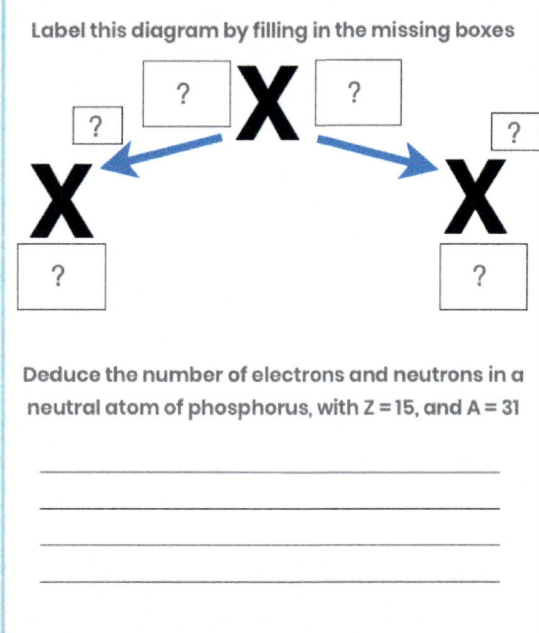

Deduce the number of electrons and neutrons in a neutral atom of phosphorus, with Z = 15, and A = 31

_____
_____
_____

Label this diagram by filling in the missing boxes

loss of electron → X^+ Cation
gain of electron → X^- Anion

Deduce the number of electrons and neutrons in a neutral atom of phosphorus, with Z = 15, and A = 31

Phosphorus has 15 protons, as Z = 15. Therefore, it must have 15 electrons to balance out against the charge of the protons, as it is a neutral atom.
31 (mass number) − 15 (protons) = 16 neutrons

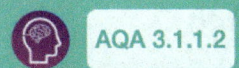

Element Isotopes

Isotopes are atoms of the same element with different number of neutrons. This means the isotopes have different mass numbers but the atomic number stays the same.

Physical properties of isotopes are different. Isotopes can have varying physical properties, because *mass* determines physical properties such as density, boiling and melting point.

Chemical properties of isotopes are pretty similar. Chemical properties are determined by the number and arrangement of electrons which do not change.

Example: Chlorine-35 and Chlorine-37 have the same number of protons (and electrons), but have a different number of neutrons. Therefore the mass number is different. They are both the same element, so have the same atomic number.

	Atomic Number	Mass Number	Protons	Electrons	Neutrons
Cl-35	17	35	17	17	18
Cl-37	17	37	17	17	20

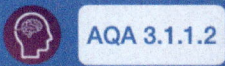

Element Isotopes

What is an isotope?

_____
_____
_____
_____
_____

What are the differences and similarities between isotopes?

_____
_____
_____
_____
_____

What is an isotope?

Isotopes are atoms of the same element but with different numbers of neutrons. Isotopes have different mass numbers but the same atomic number.

What are the differences and similarities between isotopes?

Their physical properties are different as mass determines density, boiling point and melting point. Chemical properties stay similar, as they are determined by the number of electrons, which remains the same.

A Level Geography Study Buddy

A Level Geography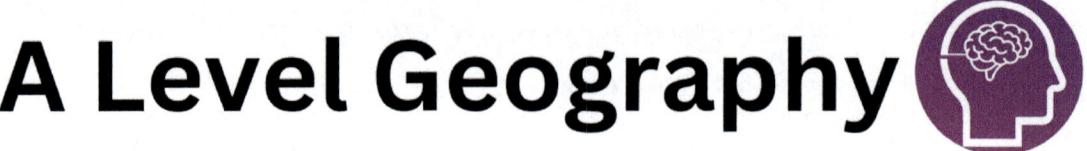

Top tips for revising each section of the AQA A Level Geography exam

Physical Geography

Water and Carbon Cycle

1. Make sure you understand the difference between surface water and groundwater – they are not interchangeable!
2. Know where the main rivers in the UK are located and be able to label them on a map.
3. Understand how river discharge is calculated, as this will likely come up in an exam question.
4. Have a good grasp of what causes floods, both man-made and natural ones.
5. Be aware of different policies that have been put in place regarding water resources, such as abstraction limits.

Hot Desert Systems and Landscapes

1. Understand how hot deserts form, including the role of latitude, altitude and local topography.
2. Study the main physical features of hot deserts, such as sand dunes and oases.
3. Be familiar with the rainfall patterns in hot desert regions and how this influences plant life (or lack thereof).
4. Learn about some of the unique animals that have adapted to survive in these conditions e.g. camels & kangaroo rats .
5 Finally, think about human activity in relation to hot deserts – why do people live there despite the harsh conditions? What are some of the challenges they face?

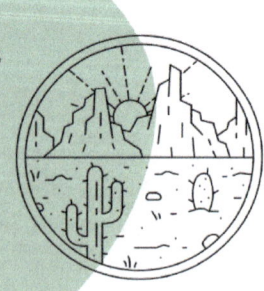

Coastal Systems and Landscapes

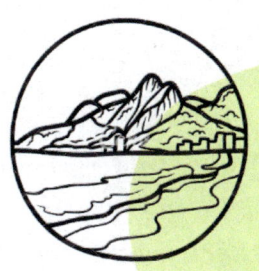

1. Understand the processes that shape coastlines including erosion, transportation and deposition.
2. Be aware of the different types of coastline – cliffed, wave-cut platform, estuarine, barrier island and delta.
3. Know how human activity can impact coasts through tourism, sea level change and coastal defence schemes.
4. Understand what landforms are created by these processes such as bays, headlands, beaches (including spit), stacks and arches.
5 Finally revise key case studies for each process e.g. Holderness for longshore drift, Dorset coast for Coastal erosion etc.

Glacial Systems and Landscapes

1. Make sure you understand the key terms associated with this topic, such as glacial period, ice age and interglacial periods.
2. Understand the processes that occur during glaciation, including abrasion, plucking and frost shattering.
3. Be able to identify different types of glaciers (e.g., Alpine glaciers) and know how they are formed.
4. Have a good understanding of past ice ages – when they occurred and what impact they had on Earth.
5. Study examples of glacial landscapes around the world (e.g. Fiords in Norway or Moraines in New Zealand).

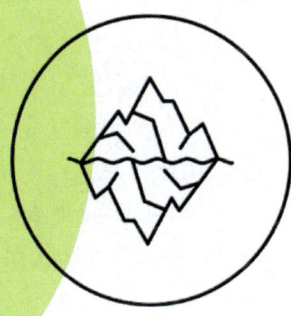

Hazards

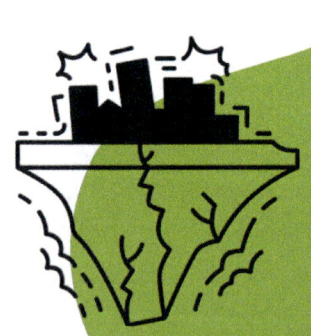

1. Make sure you are familiar with the different types of hazards that can occur. The main ones that will be covered in the exam are storms, floods, earthquakes and volcanoes.
2. Understand how each hazard forms and what conditions are needed for it to happen. For example, an earthquake is caused by movement of tectonic plates beneath the Earth's surface.
3. Know about case studies for each type of hazard so you can apply your knowledge to real-world examples. An important one to know would be the eruption of Mount Vesuvius in 79 AD which destroyed Pompeii and Herculaneum.
4. Be aware of current affairs relating to natural disasters as they could come up in questions on Paper 2 (the human geography paper). For example, there have been several large hurricanes in recent such as Hurricane Irma which hit parts of Florida in 2017.
5. Use revision websites or apps like Quizlet to test yourself on key facts and make flashcards if necessary.

Ecosystems under Stress

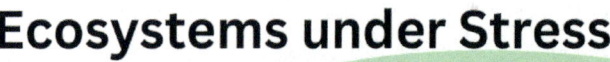

1. Make sure you understand the key terms associated with this topic, such as 'habitat fragmentation' and 'biodiversity'.
2. Be able to explain how human activities can cause ecosystems to come under stress, for example through deforestation or pollution.
3. Understand the consequences of ecosystem stress, such as a loss in biodiversity or reductions in populations of plants and animals.
4. Learn about some examples of where ecosystems are currently under stress around the world, including rainforests and coral reefs.
5 Finally, think about what measures could be taken to reduce stresses on ecosystems.

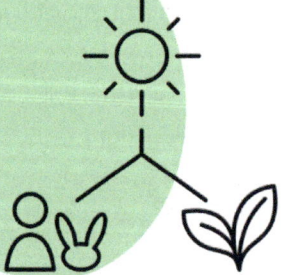

Human Geography

Global Systems and Global Governance

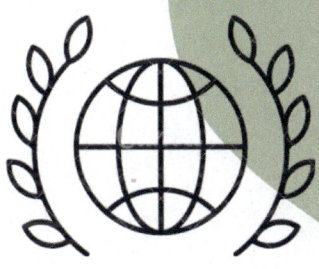

1. Understand the main global systems, including the political system, economic system and social system.
2. Be able to explain how these systems interact with each other.
3. Understand key concepts such as globalization, development and sustainability.
4. Be aware of different perspectives on global issues (e.g. North-South divide).
5 Know about important international organisations and their roles in addressing global problems (e.g. WTO, UN).

Changing Places

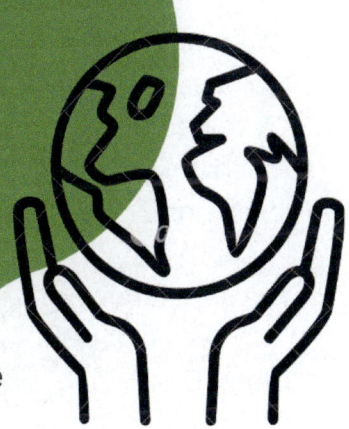

1. Make sure you know the key terms and concepts associated with each topic – this will help you to understand the question requirements and identify relevant information in your revision materials.
2. Try to relate the topics covered in this section to real-world examples, as this will make them easier to remember and apply come exam time.
3. Understand how human activity can impact on physical processes, both positively and negatively, as many questions will focus on these interactions.
4. Be able to evaluate different case studies from around the world – think about how various factors have influenced settlement patterns or caused environmental change, for example.
5. Finally, don't forget that much of the content in this section is interrelated – so revise holistically where possible!

Contemporary Urban Environments

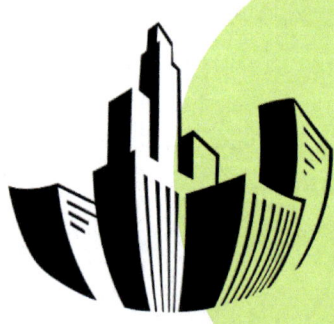

1. Understand the key terms associated with this topic, such as 'gentrification', 'urban regeneration' and 'sustainability'.
2. Be able to identify and explain different types of urban problems, including those relating to housing, transport and pollution.
3. Know a range of policy responses that have been implemented in order to tackle these issues, both at national and local level.
4. Understand how globalisation has impacted upon cities - for example, through the growth of the service sector or international investment in property
5. Be familiar with a selection of case studies from around the world which illustrate different aspects of contemporary urban life.

Population and the Environment

1. Make sure you understand the different types of population pyramids and what they represent.
2. Know how to calculate population density and be able to interpret data on maps showing this information.
3. Understand the factors that affect global populations, such as fertility rates, life expectancy and migration patterns.
4 Learn about demographic transitions and their impact on populations around the world.
5. Have an understanding of carrying capacity and its limitations.

Resource Security

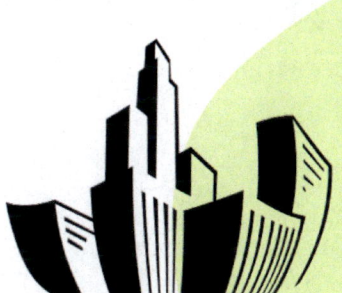

1. Make sure you understand the key terms and concepts associated with resource security, including carrying capacity, TFRs and ecological footprints.
2. Understand how different factors can impact on resource availability, such as population growth, economic development and environmental change.
3. Be able to identify case studies of countries that have experienced problems with resource insecurity, such as water shortages in Cape Town or food insecurity in Ethiopia.
4. Know about some of the measures that have been taken to address resource insecurity issues, such as desalination plants or irrigation schemes.
5. Consider the ethical implications of using resources from other parts of the world or from future generations.

Dentistry Interview Questions

100 questions to help you prepare for your dentistry interview.

Motivation for Dentistry

This is a favourite subject for dental schools, and frequently they will have an interviewer who will question you for 5 minutes straight about "why dentistry"! Here are some essential questions about other fields of research and dentistry's multidisciplinary nature. Why do you want to do dentistry?

1. What are the pros and cons of dentistry?

2. What do you want to specialise in?

3. Why would you work in a dental practice?

4. Do you have any insight into the field of dentistry?

5. Why would you want to be a dentist in a hospital?

6. What do you wish to achieve in your career in dentistry, aside from clinical practice?

7. Describe some health professionals that work alongside dentists, and explain what they do.

8. What do nurses do?

9. Why do you want to be a dentist rather than a nurse?

10. Describe an interesting dental development in recent times.

11. What extracurricular activities have you done relating to science and dentistry?

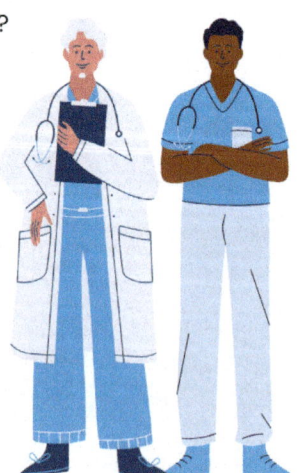

12. Discuss an interesting project, talk or article you have come across recently.
13. What are the key qualities a good dentist should have?
14. What are some of the challenges of being a dentist?
15. Do you read any dental publications?
16. Who do you consider to be the most important member of the dental team?
17. What do you know about the changing technologies in dentistry? Which do you think will have the biggest impact?
18. How much do you think dentistry impacts the patient's wider quality of life?
19. Can you tell us about any particular life experiences that you think may help or hinder you in a career in dentistry?
20. How would you dissuade someone from going into dentistry?
21. When you think about becoming a dentist, what do you look forward to most and least.
22. What impact do you hope to make in the field of dentistry?

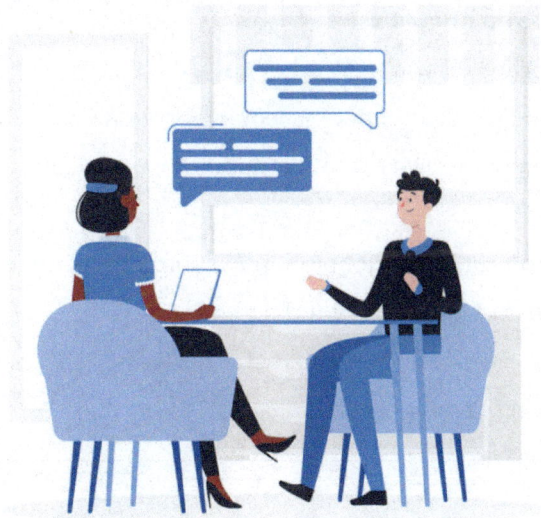

Personality

Here, you will discover how to demonstrate your empathy, compassion, and organisational skills, characteristics that will make you a great dentist. What ways of working and studying have you developed that you think will assist you through dental school? What will you need to improve?

1. How do you think you will cope with criticism from colleagues or other health professionals?
2. Is there such a thing as positive criticism?
3. What are your outside interests and hobbies? How do these complement you as a person? Which do you think you will continue at university?
4. Tell us two personal qualities you have which would make you a good dentist, and two personal shortcomings which you think you would like to overcome as you become a dentist?
5. Dental training is long and being a dentist can be stressful. Some dentists who qualify never practice. What makes you think you will stick to it?
6. What do you think are your priorities in your own personal development?
7. What qualities do you lack that would be useful for a dentist, and what do you intend to do about this?
8. What qualities do you think other people value in you?
9. How do you think other people would describe you?
10. Which of your qualities do other people find frustrating? What might you do about this?
11. You will probably have got high marks throughout school. On this dental course, most marks are awarded as 'satisfactory' or not. How will you feel about seeming 'average' in this new situation?

12. How will you cope with the death of a patient as a result of your mistakes?
13. Think of a time when you had to say 'sorry' to someone. How did that change your relationship with that person?
14. Some people are always very certain that what they believe is right. Some people are never certain. What kind of person are you in this regard?
15. What makes a good working relationship?
16. Give us an example of something about which you used to hold strong opinions but have had to change your mind. What made you change?
17. Thinking about your membership of a team (in a work, sport, school or other setting), can you tell us about the most important contributions you made to the team?
18. Tell us about a group activity you have organised. What went well and what went badly? What did you learn from it?
19. Which quality required for dentistry do you feel that you need to work on most?
20. Do you feel that your academic and scientific skills, or your people skills are more important for dentistry?
21. What are the key things to remember when talking to someone with a different viewpoint? (e.g., a patient who does not believe that they require treatment)

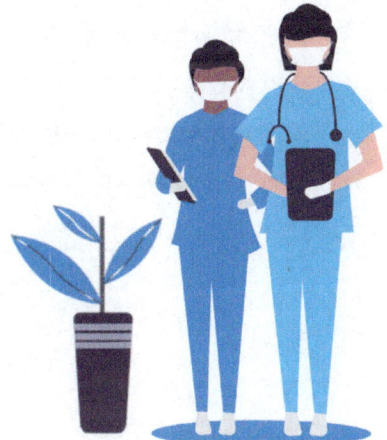

Work Experience

Whatever work experience you have undertaken, make sure to use the following questions as a guide.

1. In your work experience, what skills have you learnt that you can apply to dentistry?
2. What aspect of your work experience did you find the most challenging, and why?
3. What do you think would be the advantages, and difficulties, for a person with a major physical disability (e.g., blindness) wishing to become a dentist?
4. What have you done on work experience/inemployment previously? What would you change about what you saw, if you could, and how would you set about?
5. Thinking of your work experience, can you tell me about a difficult situation you have dealt with and what you learned from it?
6. What impressed you most about the dentists in your work experience?
7. What aspect of your work experience would you recommend to a friend thinking about dentistry, and why?
8. Reflect on what you have seen of hospitals or a healthcare environment. What would you most like to organise differently, and why?
9. Can you give me an example of how you coped with a conflict with a colleague or friend; what strategy did you use and why?
10. How did you find the fact that dentists only get 10 minutes per consultation?

11. What are the challenges of being a dentist?
12. Do you feel that the public's perception of dentists is misrepresentative?
13. What did you notice about the skills dentists needed when they were carrying out a patient history?
14. What did you notice about the dentists you were shadowing in their approach to patients?
15. During the dentist's conversations with patients, do you think that there was anything that they could improve?
16. How did patients tend to react to bad news? How would you manage this?
17. Did you witness any procedures that did not go to plan? How did the dental team cope with this?
18. What did you learn from your work experience in the dental hospital?
19. What is the difference between NHS and Private Dentistry?
20. What did you learn from your work experience in the orthodontic clinic?

The NHS

Knowing how the NHS functions and how it fits into dentistry is crucial for dental applicants. Recent years have seen a number of contentious issues, including the sugar tax and labour's proposal to eliminate Band 1 therapy.

1. What do you know about the traffic light system, and what are your opinions on it?
2. What are your thoughts on the recent sugar tax?
3. What are some alternatives of the sugar tax?
4. How should money be invested into dentistry for the NHS?
5. Should dental treatment be free on the NHS?
6. What changes have there been in dentistry over the past 100 years?
7. What are the differences between private and NHS Dentistry?
8. What are some of the reasons patients choose private treatment for their teeth over NHS?
9. Should dental treatment be free for patients on the NHS?
10. Give differences between the NHS systems in different countries in the UK
11. What is an NHS trust and how do they work?
12. Could you talk me through what would qualify as a Band 3 treatment?
13. What are your thoughts on the current NHS Dental Contract and the system of Units of Dental Activity?
14. How do price bands work for treatment under the NHS?
15. When would a dental appointment be free, even when patients are not exempt?
16. Who qualifies for free dental treatment?

Dental Conditions

It is crucial to be aware of certain dental diseases because, even if you have mentioned them in your personal statement, interviewers may still ask you questions about them on the actual interview day.

1. Why do some people underestimate the value of their teeth?
2. As well as undervaluing their teeth, many can't access dental care. Why is this?
3. What do you know about gum disease?
4. What do you know about how diabetes affects the teeth?
5. What do you know about oral cancer?
6. What do you know about preventative dentistry?
7. Could you tell me a little more about root canal treatment?
8. What do you know about amalgam?
9. One of the biggest problems to to teeth is smoking. What do you know about this?
10. Do you think we should ban tobacco in the UK?
11. What are the differences between composite and amalgam?
12. What is a crown and what are they made of?
13. What determines the survival of a tooth?
14. Should tobacco be banned?
15. What can be done if a tooth has died?
16. Do you think the cultural attitude towards dentition has changed?
17. How does alcohol affect the oral cavity?
18. Give risk factors for oral cancer
19. Describe how you would tell a patient that their tooth needs to be extracted.

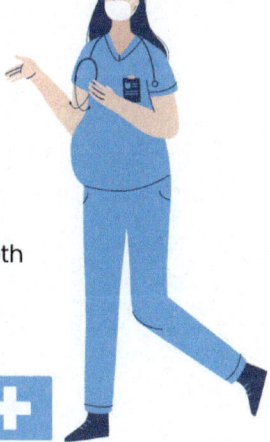

www.medicmind.co.uk

Printed in Great Britain
by Amazon